CARB CYCLING FOR BEGINNERS

Master Metabolism and Transform Your Body with Tasty, Energizing Low-Carb & High-Carb Recipes. Lose Fat, Build Muscle and Boost Energy

Marco Ferrari

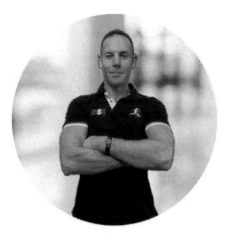

Marco Ferrari is a Personal Trainer Certified by ISSA (International Science Sport Association).

Disclaimer Notice:

The information contained within this document is for educational and entertainment purposes only. All effort has been executed to present accurate, up to date, and reliable, complete information. No warranties of any kind are declared or implied.

Readers acknowledge that the author is not engaging in the rendering of legal, financial, medical or professional advice. Anyone who decides to put this advice into practice does so with responsibility for their own choices and with awareness of the risks involved in sporting practices.

Under no circumstances will any blame or legal responsibility be held against the publisher, or author, for any damages, reparation, or monetary loss due to the information contained within this book.

Table of Contents

❈ HERE IS YOUR FREE GIFT!

SCAN HERE TO DOWNLOAD IT

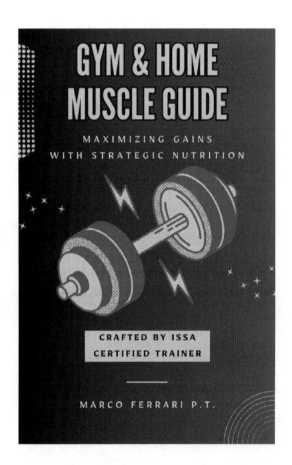

Inside this guide, you'll discover:

• **Comprehensive Training Strategies**: Unlock the secrets to effective muscle gains with dual-environment workout plans, optimizing your fitness whether you're in the gym or at home.

• **Nutritional Synergy**: Discover how to align your diet with your workout regimen for maximum muscle growth and fat loss, using proven nutritional tactics tailored to your body's needs.

• **Adaptable for All Levels**: Whether you're a beginner or an advanced athlete, find detailed guidance for every stage of your fitness journey, complete with strategies for progression and success.

And so much more...

SCAN HERE TO DOWNLOAD IT

PART 1: UNDERSTANDING CARB CYCLING

Chapter 1: Introduction

Have you ever thought about comparing your metabolism to a blazing fire? Just as a fire thrives on the right fuel to intensify its heat, your metabolism operates at its best when fueled with the right ingredients. Failing to supply ample fuel over an extended period can result in the gradual weakening and eventual sputtering out of your metabolic "flames."

In the quest for rapid weight loss, carb cycling, a dietary approach involving strategic variations in carbohydrate intake, emerges as a promising strategy. This method, characterized by consuming higher amounts of carbs on specific days of the week, stimulates digestive and metabolic processes crucial for effective weight management. The art of consuming carbohydrates in adequate quantities at precise times acts as a reset for your "metabolic thermostat." This signals the body to produce essential hormones such as leptin and thyroid hormones, regulating appetite and sustaining a heightened metabolism. Nevertheless, it's crucial to strike a balance, as excessive carb consumption can lead to unintended weight gain.

What sets carb cycling apart from other diet plans is its targeted increase in carbohydrate intake, coupled with potential variations in calorie consumption, strategically timed to optimize metabolic function. Unlike some restrictive and overwhelming long-term diet plans, carb cycling proves to be a more adaptable and manageable approach, fitting seamlessly into busy schedules.

What is Carb Cycling?

It is a dietary strategy involving periodic elevation of carbohydrate intake on specific days, contrasted with lower carb consumption on alternate days, facilitating more accessible weight loss. Essentially, adhering to a carb cycling meal plan means incorporating adequate amounts of unprocessed and nutrient-dense carbs every other day or at intervals aligned with individual goals.

Widely embraced by bodybuilders, fitness models, and various athletes, carb cycling taps into the unique role of carbohydrates as the body's primary fuel source. Carbohydrates swiftly convert into glucose and glycogen, powering cells and generating ATP (energy). Your metabolism fluctuates based on calorie and macronutrient intake, with studies highlighting the positive impact of sufficient carb consumption on both prolonged, low-intensity and short, high-intensity exercises. Additionally, controlled carb intake aids in appetite regulation, enhances satiety, and prevents prolonged feelings of deprivation.

While the specifics of each carb cycling plan may vary based on individual goals, a common feature is the inclusion of one to three days per week for increased consumption of carb-rich foods, such as potatoes or grains. On lower-carb days, the foundation of meals comprises non-starchy vegetables, grass-fed meats, eggs, and healthy fats.

Some carb cycling plans even incorporate a "cheat day" for indulging in decadent foods, serving as a guilt-free reward for commitment to the dietary regimen. In essence, carb cycling offers a flexible and effective approach to managing weight and optimizing metabolic performance.

Chapter 2: Foundations of Carb Cycling

Carb cycling is a dietary approach that entails rotating between days of high and low carbohydrate consumption throughout the week. Unlike diets that completely eliminate carbs, carb cycling encourages adjusting your carb intake based on your daily activity level, either increasing or reducing it accordingly.

The Science and Mechanism

Understanding the mechanics behind carb cycling is key to unlocking its potential benefits. Carb cycling is a dietary strategy that involves purposeful variations in carbohydrate intake to influence metabolic processes and improve overall well-being. This approach relies on a flexible adjustment of macronutrient consumption to cater to individual needs, recognizing the dynamic relationship between these nutrients and the body's energy requirements.

Carbohydrates, serving as a primary energy source, play a central role in the science of carb cycling. By strategically manipulating the intake of these macronutrients, carb cycling seeks to optimize metabolic functions, promoting a more efficient energy utilization process within the body.

The primary objective of carb cycling is to harness the unique properties of carbohydrates in fueling cellular activities. Upon consumption, carbohydrates undergo breakdown into glucose, serving as an immediate energy source for the body. Any surplus glucose is transformed into glycogen and stored in the muscles and liver, serving as a reserve to meet increased energy demands when necessary.

The cyclical nature of carb cycling involves alternating periods of higher and lower carbohydrate intake. During phases of increased carb consumption, the body experiences a surge in blood glucose levels, prompting the release of insulin. The pancreas produces insulin, a hormone that plays a crucial role in facilitating the uptake of glucose by cells, ultimately supporting energy production. This process not only replenishes glycogen stores but also promotes an anabolic state, crucial for muscle growth and repair.

Conversely, during low-carb phases, the body relies on alternative fuel sources, such as stored fat. As carbohydrate intake decreases, insulin levels drop, signaling the body to switch to fat metabolism. This transition encourages the breakdown of stored fat into ketone bodies, which serve as an alternative energy source. By cycling between these phases, carb cycling aims to strike a balance between utilizing immediate energy from carbohydrates and tapping into stored fat for sustained fuel.

The dynamic interplay between carbohydrates and insulin also influences other key hormones, such as leptin and ghrelin, which regulate appetite and hunger. When carbohydrate intake is strategically increased, leptin levels rise, signaling satiety to the brain and curbing appetite. On the contrary, lower carbohydrate phases may result in decreased leptin levels, potentially intensifying hunger signals.[1,2]

Moreover, carb cycling can positively impact thyroid hormones, contributing to enhanced metabolic rate. Thyroid hormones play a crucial role in regulating the body's metabolism by influencing energy expenditure and heat production. By modulating carbohydrate intake, carb cycling seeks to optimize thyroid function, promoting a more responsive and efficient metabolism.

Health and Fitness Benefits

Delving into the world of carb cycling reveals a host of benefits that extend beyond the realm of metabolism. This dietary strategy, characterized by strategic variations in carbohydrate intake, offers a versatile approach to achieving health and fitness goals. Let's unravel the layers of advantages associated with carb cycling.

1. Weight Management: One of the primary draws of carb cycling lies in its potential to support effective weight management. The cyclical nature of this approach prevents the body from adapting to a constant calorie intake, fostering a more dynamic environment for fat loss. By strategically alternating between high and low-carb phases, individuals may experience enhanced fat loss while preserving valuable lean muscle mass. This makes carb cycling an attractive option for those seeking a sustainable and efficient strategy for weight control.

2. Preservation of Lean Muscle Mass: Unlike traditional diets that may lead to muscle loss along with fat, carb cycling prioritizes the preservation of lean muscle mass. During high-carb phases, the body is supplied with ample energy to fuel workouts and support muscle growth. This emphasis on maintaining muscle mass contributes to a more toned and sculpted physique, distinguishing carb cycling from approaches that may compromise overall body composition.

3. Improved Athletic Performance: Carb cycling has found favor among athletes and fitness enthusiasts due to its positive impact on performance. Carbohydrates are the body's preferred energy source, especially during high-intensity exercises. By strategically timing higher carbohydrate intake, individuals engaging in a variety of physical activities, from prolonged, low-intensity workouts to short, high-intensity bursts, may experience improved endurance and sustained performance levels. This adaptability makes carb cycling a valuable tool for optimizing athletic achievements.

4. Balanced Blood Sugar Levels: Maintaining stable blood sugar levels is crucial for overall health, and carb cycling can play a role in achieving this balance. During low-carb phases, the body relies on alternative fuel sources, such as stored fat, helping to prevent rapid spikes and crashes in blood sugar. The strategic inclusion of higher-carb days provides a controlled influx of glucose, preventing prolonged periods of low blood sugar and promoting a more balanced and sustainable energy supply.

5. Hormonal Regulation: Carb cycling influences key hormones involved in appetite control and metabolic rate. The interplay between carbohydrate intake and insulin levels impacts hormones like leptin and ghrelin, which play vital roles in regulating hunger and satiety. By strategically adjusting carbohydrate consumption, individuals can modulate these hormonal responses, promoting a more balanced appetite and potentially supporting long-term weight management.

6. Enhanced Metabolic Rate: Beyond hormonal regulation, carb cycling may contribute to a more responsive metabolism. Thyroid hormones, critical for regulating metabolic functions, can be positively influenced by the modulation of carbohydrate intake. This optimization of thyroid function supports an efficient metabolism, potentially aiding in energy expenditure and promoting overall metabolic health.

7. Psychological Well-Being: The psychological benefits of carb cycling, including its flexibility and positive impact on mental well-being, are explored in greater detail in the following section.

Psychological Benefits

Carb cycling, as a dietary strategy characterized by strategic shifts in carbohydrate intake, extends its impact beyond the physical realm, offering a host of psychological benefits. Understanding the interplay between carb cycling and mental well-being reveals how this approach can positively influence attitudes towards food, adherence to dietary plans, and overall satisfaction with a healthier lifestyle.

1. Flexible Approach to Eating: One of the key psychological benefits of carb cycling lies in its inherent flexibility. Traditional diets often come with rigid rules and restrictions, leading to a sense of confinement. Carb cycling, with its cyclical nature, allows individuals to navigate through periods of both higher and lower carbohydrate intake. This flexibility provides a sense of control over one's eating patterns, reducing the feeling of being tethered to a stringent dietary regimen.

2. Variety in Food Choices: Carb cycling encourages a diverse range of food choices by incorporating different types of carbohydrates during high-carb phases. This variety not only caters to nutritional needs but also adds a flavorful dimension to meals. Enjoying a spectrum of foods, from nutrient-dense carbohydrates to wholesome fats and proteins, can contribute to a more satisfying and enjoyable eating experience.

3. Avoidance of Dietary Monotony: The cyclical nature of carb cycling helps individuals steer clear of the monotony often associated with prolonged dietary restrictions. By incorporating higher-carb days or even designated "cheat days," carb cycling introduces a break from the routine, preventing feelings of deprivation. This intentional break contributes to a more positive relationship with food, reducing the risk of burnout and promoting sustained adherence to the dietary plan.

4. Positive Reinforcement and Rewards: Many carb cycling plans include the concept of "cheat days" or indulgent meals strategically placed within the cycle. These moments serve as positive reinforcements and rewards for adhering to the dietary plan. By allowing occasional indulgences without guilt, carb cycling recognizes the importance of balance and moderation. This positive reinforcement can contribute to a healthier mindset towards food and dietary choices, fostering a positive mindset towards long-term lifestyle changes.

5. Reduced Feelings of Deprivation: Traditional diets often instill a sense of deprivation, leading to cravings and potential deviations from the plan. Carb cycling, with its intentional inclusion of higher-carb phases, mitigates these feelings of deprivation. The ability to enjoy favorite carbohydrate-rich foods during specific periods reduces the psychological stress associated with strict dietary restrictions, making the overall experience more sustainable and enjoyable.

6. Cognitive Break from Calorie Counting: Controlling calories and calorie balance, daily and weekly, is necessary in the diet, however, this can be mentally taxing. Carb cycling can offers a cognitive break from constant calorie monitoring, especially during higher-carb phases. While still emphasizing mindful eating, the cyclical nature allows individuals to focus on the nutritional quality of their food rather than becoming fixated on exact calorie counts, promoting a healthier and more relaxed approach to eating.

7. Sustainable Lifestyle Integration: Carb cycling, with its adaptable and sustainable approach, lends itself well to integration into various lifestyles. The psychological benefit of adopting a dietary strategy that aligns with personal preferences and schedules contributes to long-term adherence. This adaptability makes carb cycling a more feasible and sustainable option for those seeking lasting improvements in their eating habits and overall well-being.

Chapter 3: Setting Up for Success

Goal Setting and Personal Assessment

Starting a carb cycling routine involves setting personalized goals and conducting a thorough self-assessment. By understanding your individual objectives, assessing your current habits, and tailoring your approach accordingly, you can optimize the effectiveness of carb cycling for your unique needs.

- **Establishing Clear Goals:** Before diving into carb cycling, it's crucial to define your specific health and fitness goals. Whether you aim to lose weight, build muscle, enhance athletic performance, or improve overall well-being, establishing clear objectives provides a roadmap for your carb cycling journey. Your goals will influence the duration, intensity, and structure of your carb cycling plan, ensuring it aligns with your desired outcomes.

- **Conducting a Personal Assessment:** Conducting a thorough self-assessment involves taking stock of your current dietary habits, activity levels, and overall lifestyle. This reflective process provides valuable insights into areas that may need adjustment and helps identify patterns that can impact the success of your carb cycling plan. Assess your current carbohydrate intake, meal timing, and the types of foods you regularly consume to form a baseline for making informed adjustments.

- **Determining Carb Tolerance:** Understanding your body's response to carbohydrates is a crucial aspect of personalizing your carb cycling approach. Carb tolerance varies among individuals, and factors such as metabolism, activity level, and insulin sensitivity play key roles. Experimenting with different carbohydrate intake levels during specific phases of carb cycling allows you to determine the optimal amount that supports your goals without unwanted side effects, such as energy crashes or excessive weight gain.

- **Tailoring the Plan to Your Lifestyle:** One of the strengths of carb cycling lies in its adaptability to different lifestyles. Consider your daily routine, work schedule, and social commitments when designing your carb cycling plan. Tailoring the plan to seamlessly integrate with your lifestyle enhances its sustainability. Choose carb cycling intervals that align with your preferences, making it easier to adhere to the dietary strategy over the long term.

- **Identifying Trigger Foods and Cravings:** Recognizing trigger foods and understanding your cravings is essential for successful carb cycling. Identify foods that may lead to overconsumption or derail your progress. This awareness enables you to make informed choices during higher-carb phases and navigate potential challenges. By incorporating strategies to manage cravings, such as choosing nutrient-dense alternatives, you can maintain control over your dietary choices.

- **Tracking Progress and Adjusting Goals:** Regularly tracking your progress is a vital component of goal setting in carb cycling. Monitor changes in weight, body composition, energy levels, and overall well-being. Use this data to adjust your goals and fine-tune your carb cycling plan as needed. Celebrate achievements and be open to modifications that better align with your evolving objectives.

- **Balancing Macronutrients:** Carb cycling is not solely about manipulating carbohydrate intake; it also involves balancing other macronutrients—proteins and fats. Assess your current protein and fat consumption and ensure they align with your goals. Protein is essential for muscle repair and growth, while healthy fats contribute to overall well-being. Striking the right balance ensures a comprehensive approach to your nutritional needs.

- **Incorporating Variety and Nutrient Density:** A well-rounded carb cycling plan includes a variety of nutrient-dense foods. Ensure your diet incorporates a colorful array of fruits, vegetables, lean proteins, and whole grains. This diversity not only provides essential vitamins and minerals but also contributes to the overall enjoyment of your meals. Experiment with different food combinations to maintain interest and satisfaction in your dietary choices.

• **Allowing for Flexibility:** While structure is crucial in carb cycling, allowing for flexibility is equally important. Life is dynamic, and unforeseen circumstances may arise. Be prepared to adapt your carb cycling plan when needed, without feeling discouraged. A flexible mindset promotes resilience, making it easier to navigate challenges and maintain a positive relationship with your dietary journey.

• **Seeking Professional Guidance if Needed:** If you find the process overwhelming or if you have specific health concerns, consider seeking guidance from a healthcare professional or a registered dietitian. They can provide personalized advice, address any potential risks, and ensure that your carb cycling plan aligns with your individual health profile.

Calculating TDEE and Macronutrients

Calculating TDEE

Determining your Total Daily Energy Expenditure (TDEE) is a crucial process to comprehend the number of calories required for your body to sustain its present weight. TDEE considers both your Basal Metabolic Rate (BMR) and your daily level of activity. Here's a simple guide to help you calculate your TDEE:

1. **Determine Your Basal Metabolic Rate (BMR)**

Using the Harris-Benedict Equation (revised)

For Men: BMR = 88.362 + (13.397 × weight in kg) + (4.799 × height in cm) - (5.677 × age in years)

For Women: BMR = 447.593 + (9.247 × weight in kg) + (3.098 × height in cm) - (4.330 × age in years)

Example for a woman:

- Age: 30 years
- Weight: 65 kg
- Height: 160 cm

BMR = 447.593 + (9.247 × 65) + (3.098 × 160) - (4.330 × 30)
= 447.593 + 600.955 + 494.880 - 129.900
= 1413.528 calories per day

Using the Katch-McArdle Equation. If you know your lean body mass, this equation provides an alternative method of calculating BMR, offering guidance appropriate to your body composition. This can lead to a more accurate estimate of BMR.

(21.6 x LBM) + 370

LBM = lean body mass in kg

Example for a men:

- Weight: 80 kg
- Body Fat: 15%
- LBM: 80 − 15% = 65 Kg

BMR = (21,6 x 65) + 370 = 1774 calories per day

2. **Factor in Your Activity Level**

Your TDEE is not just your BMR; it also considers your daily activity level. Different multipliers are used based on how active you are:

- Sedentary (little to no exercise): TDEE = BMR × 1.2
- Lightly active (light exercise/sports 1-3 days/week): TDEE = BMR × 1.375

- Moderately active (moderate exercise/sports 3-5 days/week): TDEE = BMR × 1.55
- Very active (hard exercise/sports 6-7 days a week): TDEE = BMR × 1.725
- Extremely active (very hard exercise/sports & physical job or 2x training): TDEE = BMR × 1.9

For our example, if the person engages in moderate exercise 3-5 days a week, the TDEE would be:

TDEE = 1413.528 × 1.55 = 2191.3734 calories per day

3. **Set Your Goals**

Once you have your TDEE, you can set specific goals based on your objectives:

- **Weight Loss:** Aim for a calorie intake 15-20% below your TDEE.
- **Muscle Gain:** Aim for a calorie intake 5-10% above your TDEE.
- **Maintenance:** Aim to match your TDEE for weight maintenance.

Remember to always stick to your daily and weekly calorie balance.

4. **Adjust as Needed**

The determined Total Daily Energy Expenditure (TDEE) serves as an approximation, with individual elements like metabolism and lifestyle potentially impacting your specific calorie requirements. Keep track of your advancements and modify your calorie consumption accordingly, considering your body's responses.

5. **Consider Macronutrient Distribution**

While TDEE provides your total calorie needs, understanding the distribution of macronutrients (proteins, carbohydrates, and fats) is crucial. Depending on your goals, you may adjust the percentages of these macronutrients within your daily calorie intake.

Macronutrients

Understanding the role of macronutrients is paramount when diving into the world of carb cycling. Macronutrients, commonly known as "macros," include proteins, carbohydrates, and fats. These nutrients form the foundation of your diet, and manipulating their intake is a key aspect of effective carb cycling. Let's explore the significance of each macronutrient, how they contribute to the carb cycling approach, and how you can tailor your intake to meet your specific health and fitness goals.

Proteins

Proteins are fundamental to the body's structure and function, serving as the building blocks for muscles, tissues, enzymes, and hormones. In the context of carb cycling, proteins play a crucial role in supporting muscle maintenance, repair, and growth.

- **Daily Protein Intake:** Daily Protein Intake: The recommended protein intake varies based on individual factors such as activity level, age, diet, and goals. Generally, a range of 0.93 to 1.2 gm of protein per kg of body weight is considered suitable for sedentary adult humans[3]. For the sports population, especially those training in strength and power disciplines like resistance training, protein requirements are significantly higher, and they should consume about twice as much. Thus, a protein intake of between 1.6 and 2 g per kg of body weight is generally recommended, especially to preserve muscle mass. During periods of calorie restriction, protein intake can be slightly increased to between 2.3 and 3.1 g of protein per kg of Lean Body Mass[4].

- **High-Carb and Low-Carb Days**: Although carbohydrate intakes fluctuate during the carb cycling week, the amount of protein should remain stable regardless of whether it's high carb or low carb day.

Carbohydrates

Carbohydrates serve as the body's primary and preferred energy source, providing the fuel needed for physical and mental activities. In carb cycling, manipulating carbohydrate intake on different days influences energy availability and supports specific metabolic goals.

- **Daily Carbohydrate Intake:** The amount of carbohydrates you consume daily varies based on your goals, activity level, and overall calorie needs. Ideally, on low-carb days, the intake should be in the range of 1-2 gm per kg of body weight. On high-carb days, it can increase to 4-6 gm per kg of body weight. In any case, carbohydrate intake should meet or slightly exceed the TDEE.

- **High-Carb Days:** These days are characterized by an increased intake of complex carbohydrates, approximately 25% more, such as whole grains, fruits, and starchy vegetables. This surge in carbohydrates replenishes glycogen stores, providing a readily available energy source for intense workouts and sustaining peak performance. Significantly increase carbohydrate intake to meet or slightly exceed TDEE.

- **Low-Carb Days:** On low-carb days, the focus shifts to non-starchy vegetables, lean proteins, and healthy fats. Reducing carbohydrate intake prompts the body to utilize stored fat for energy, supporting fat loss while maintaining stable blood sugar levels.

Individuals who prefer not to track macronutrients due to varying energy expenditure or personal preference, but still wish to cycle carbohydrates, can rely on simple estimates for carbohydrate amounts. Low-carbohydrate days are defined as those with 50-150g of carbohydrates, medium days range from 150-300g, and high-carbohydrate days involve 300-500g.

Fats

Dietary fats play a crucial role in hormone production, cell structure, and the absorption of fat-soluble vitamins. Including the right types and amounts of fats in your diet is essential for overall well-being.

- **Daily Fat Intake:** Fat intake can be adjusted based on daily caloric needs, but it is generally kept moderate to low to balance the higher intake of carbs and protein. A common recommendation is about 20-30% of total daily calories. However, the range can vary from 0.5 to 1.5 gm per kg of body weight, with adjustments made on an individual basis..

- **High-Carb Days:** On high-carb days, include healthy fats such as avocados, nuts, and olive oil in moderation. These fats contribute to satiety and overall nutrient intake while supporting hormonal balance.

- **Low-Carb Days:** During low-carb days, slightly higher fat intake helps compensate for the reduced energy from carbohydrates. Emphasize sources of healthy fats, such as avocados, nuts, seeds, and fatty fish, to provide sustained energy and promote a feeling of fullness.

Adapting Macro Ratios to Your Goals

The distribution of macronutrients within your daily caloric intake can be adjusted based on your specific health and fitness goals.

- **Weight Loss:** If your primary goal is weight loss, creating a calorie deficit is essential. Focus on maintaining a balance between proteins, carbohydrates, and fats while keeping overall calorie intake below your Total Daily Energy Expenditure (TDEE).

- **Muscle Gain:** For those aiming to build muscle, a slight calorie surplus is beneficial. Ensure an adequate protein intake to support muscle growth, coupled with an increase in overall calorie intake, especially on high-carb days.

- **Maintenance:** To maintain your current weight, align your daily calorie intake with your TDEE. Maintain a balanced distribution of macronutrients to support overall health and well-being.

Monitoring and Adjusting

Regularly monitoring your progress is crucial to determine how your body responds to the macronutrient ratios during carb cycling.

- **Weight and Body Composition:** Keep track of changes in your weight and body composition over time. Adjust your macronutrient ratios based on whether you are progressing towards your goals.

- **Energy Levels and Performance:** Pay attention to your energy levels and performance during workouts. If you experience consistent fatigue on low-carb days, consider adjusting your macronutrient distribution to better suit your needs.

Staying Hydrated and Considering Micronutrients

While macronutrients are essential, don't overlook the importance of staying hydrated and ensuring an adequate intake of micronutrients (vitamins and minerals). Hydration supports overall health then helps maintain optimal bodily functions.

Chapter 4: The Carb Cycling Process

Embarking on the carb cycling journey involves a strategic and cyclical approach to carbohydrate intake. This dietary method aims to optimize energy levels, support various fitness goals, and maintain overall well-being. Understanding the intricacies of high-carb days, low-carb days, and the transitional phase to no-carb days is key to harnessing the benefits of carb cycling effectively.

High-Carb Days

High-carb days are a foundational component of carb cycling, strategically timed to provide a surge in carbohydrates that fuels energy-demanding activities. The primary goals of high-carb days include supporting intense workouts, replenishing glycogen stores, and promoting overall metabolic efficiency.

- **Carbohydrate Intake:** On high-carb days, the emphasis is on consuming a higher quantity of complex carbohydrates. Whole grains, fruits, starchy vegetables, and legumes become the primary sources of energy. Aim for a carbohydrate intake to cover your TDEE on these days.

- **Timing and Performance:** Timing is crucial on high-carb days, especially around workouts. Consuming a carbohydrate-rich meal or snack before and after exercise ensures that your body has an immediate and accessible source of energy. This supports endurance, strength, and optimal performance during training sessions[5,6,7]. Most importantly, this ensures that nutrients are more easily delivered to the muscles, rather than to the adipose tissue.

- **Glycogen Replenishment:** The increased carbohydrate intake on high-carb days serves to replenish glycogen stores in muscles and the liver. Glycogen is a form of stored energy, and maintaining adequate levels is essential for sustained physical performance.

- **Metabolic Boost:** High-carb days can provide a temporary boost to metabolism, signaling the body that it is well-fueled and encouraging efficient energy utilization. This metabolic stimulation contributes to the overall effectiveness of carb cycling in achieving various fitness goals.

Low-Carb Days

In contrast to high-carb days, low-carb days involve a reduction in carbohydrate intake, prompting the body to shift its reliance on stored fat for energy. This phase is instrumental in promoting fat utilization, supporting weight loss, and encouraging metabolic adaptation.

- **Carbohydrate Restriction:** On low-carb days, the focus is on restricting carbohydrate intake. Non-starchy vegetables, lean proteins, and healthy fats become the primary components of meals. Aim for a carbohydrate intake ranging from 0.5 to 1.0 gm per pound of body weight on these days.

- **Promoting Fat Utilization:** The intentional reduction in carbohydrates signals the body to utilize stored fat as a primary energy source. This shift encourages fat burning, contributing to weight loss and the preservation of lean muscle mass.

- **Stabilizing Blood Sugar Levels:** Lower carbohydrate intake on these days helps stabilize blood sugar levels. This prevents the rapid spikes and crashes associated with high-carb meals, promoting a more consistent and sustained energy supply.

- **Enhanced Insulin Sensitivity:** The temporary reduction in carbohydrate intake during low-carb days can enhance insulin sensitivity. Improved insulin sensitivity supports better blood sugar regulation and may have positive implications for long-term metabolic health.

Transitioning: No-Carb Days

As part of a more advanced approach to carb cycling, some individuals incorporate no-carb days into their cycling routine. These days involve an almost complete elimination of carbohydrates, challenging the body to rely on alternative fuel sources and promoting metabolic flexibility.

- **Carbohydrate Elimination:** On no-carb days, the goal is to minimize carbohydrate intake as much as possible. This often involves focusing on proteins, healthy fats, and non-starchy vegetables while avoiding traditional carbohydrate sources.

- **Ketogenic Influence:** No-carb days may induce a state of ketosis, where the body produces ketones as an alternative fuel source in the absence of carbohydrates. This metabolic state has been associated with increased fat burning and mental clarity.

- **Challenging Metabolic Adaptation:** Introducing no-carb days challenges the body's metabolic adaptability. The shift from relying on carbohydrates to utilizing fats for energy enhances the flexibility of the metabolic pathways, potentially supporting overall metabolic health.

- **Cautions and Individual Variation:** It's important to approach no-carb days cautiously and consider individual variations. Not everyone may benefit from or tolerate prolonged periods without carbohydrates. Listening to your body and consulting with a healthcare professional or nutrition expert is crucial when implementing more advanced carb cycling strategies.

Chapter 5: Exercise and Carb Cycling

Maximizing the synergy between exercise and carb cycling is a dynamic strategy that can significantly enhance the effectiveness of your fitness routine. By strategically aligning specific types of training with different phases of carb cycling, you can optimize energy utilization, support muscle development, and promote overall well-being. Let's delve into the types of training that complement high-carb days, ideal for muscle training, and low-carb days, suitable for LISS (Low-Intensity Steady State) cardio training or rest.

High-Carb Days

High-carb days provide an opportunity to capitalize on increased energy availability. The infusion of complex carbohydrates into your diet on these days serves as a potent fuel source, enabling you to engage in more demanding and intense workout sessions. Here are types of training that synergize well with high-carb days:

• **Weight Training:** High-carb days are ideal for incorporating weight training sessions. Whether using free weights, resistance machines, or engaging in bodyweight exercises, the heightened carbohydrate intake supports enhanced strength, endurance, and muscle recovery. Aim for compound movements that target multiple muscle groups, such as squats, deadlifts, bench presses, leg press, hack-squat, pull-up, Barbell Row etc. Always choose exercises that best suit your physical needs and that you feel most comfortable with.

• **High-Intensity Interval Training (HIIT):** The explosive energy provided by increased carbohydrates makes high-carb days conducive to incorporating HIIT workouts. HIIT involves short bursts of intense exercise followed by brief rest periods. This style of training not only boosts cardiovascular fitness but also contributes to calorie burning and metabolic elevation.

• **Functional Training:** Engaging in functional training exercises on high-carb days is beneficial. This includes movements that mimic real-life activities and enhance overall athleticism. Examples include kettlebell swings, medicine ball throws, TRX and agility drills. The ample carbohydrate supply supports sustained effort during these dynamic and varied exercises.

Low-Carb Days

On low-carb days, the focus shifts towards promoting fat utilization as the primary energy source. Adjusting your workout routine on these days to align with reduced carbohydrate intake allows you to capitalize on the body's inclination to burn stored fat. Consider the following types of training for low-carb days:

• **Low-Intensity Steady-State (LISS) Cardio:** LISS cardio, characterized by sustained, moderate-intensity exercise, is well-suited for low-carb days. Activities such as brisk walking, cycling, or swimming at a consistent pace encourage fat burning while minimizing reliance on immediate carbohydrate stores. LISS provides a cardiovascular benefit without the need for glycogen replenishment.

• **Yoga or Pilates:** Incorporating yoga or Pilates sessions on low-carb days promotes flexibility, balance, and core strength. These exercises, with their lower intensity, align with the energy profile of low-carb phases. Additionally, they contribute to overall well-being and may aid in recovery, especially when coupled with mindful breathing and relaxation techniques.

• **Active Recovery:** Designating low-carb days for active recovery is a prudent approach. Engage in light activities such as leisurely cycling, swimming, or gentle stretching to promote blood flow and aid in muscle recovery. Active recovery sessions contribute to maintaining mobility and preventing stiffness without placing excessive demands on carbohydrate stores.

Rest Days

While not explicitly associated with a specific carbohydrate intake, rest days play a crucial role in any fitness routine. On rest days, allowing the body to recover and repair is paramount for long-term success. Consider the following practices to optimize your rest days within the context of carb cycling:

- **Complete Rest:** On designated rest days, prioritize complete physical rest. This allows the body to recover from the stressors of previous workouts, reducing the risk of overtraining and promoting optimal muscle repair. Adequate rest contributes to sustained energy levels and prevents burnout.

- **Mindfulness and Stress Reduction:** Incorporating mindfulness practices such as meditation or deep breathing exercises on rest days contributes to overall well-being. Managing stress is integral to the recovery process, and these practices can positively impact both mental and physical aspects of health.

- **Hydration and Nutrient-Dense Foods:** Emphasize hydration and consume nutrient-dense foods on rest days. Proper hydration supports various bodily functions, including nutrient transport and waste elimination. Choosing nourishing foods ensures that your body receives essential vitamins, minerals, and antioxidants, supporting overall health.

Individualized Approach

While general guidelines can provide a framework, it's essential to listen to your body and tailor your workout routine to your individual preferences, energy levels, and responses. Everyone's body reacts differently to varying training intensities and carbohydrate intake. Pay attention to how you feel during and after workouts, adjusting the types of training and intensity based on your unique needs.

- **Feedback Mechanism:** Your body provides valuable feedback through energy levels, mood, and recovery. If you consistently feel fatigued or notice a lack of progress, reassess your training regimen and consider modifying the distribution of high-carb and low-carb days.

- **Periodization:** Implementing a form of periodization in your training plan, where you alternate between phases of higher and lower intensity, aligns with the cyclical nature of carb cycling. This approach helps prevent plateaus, enhances adaptation, and keeps your workouts dynamic.

Hydration and Post-Workout Nutrition

Regardless of the type of training or carb cycling phase, prioritizing hydration and post-workout nutrition is crucial. Proper hydration supports optimal performance and recovery, while consuming a balanced post-workout meal containing proteins and carbohydrates aids in muscle repair and replenishes glycogen stores.

References

1. Adamska-Patruno, Edyta et al. "The relationship between the leptin/ghrelin ratio and meals with various macronutrient contents in men with different nutritional status: a randomized crossover study." Nutrition journal vol. 17,1 118. 28 Dec. 2018, doi:10.1186/s12937-018-0427-x

2. Gavrieli A, Mantzoros CS. Novel Molecules Regulating Energy Homeostasis: Physiology and Regulation by Macronutrient Intake and Weight Loss. Endocrinol Metab (Seoul). 2016;31(3):361-372. doi:10.3803/EnM.2016.31.3.361

3. Elango, Rajavel et al. "Evidence that protein requirements have been significantly underestimated." Current opinion in clinical nutrition and metabolic care vol. 13,1 (2010): 52-7. doi:10.1097/MCO.0b013e328332f9b7

4. Nunes, Everson A et al. "Systematic review and meta-analysis of protein intake to support muscle mass and function in healthy adults." Journal of cachexia, sarcopenia and muscle vol. 13,2 (2022): 795-810. doi:10.1002/jcsm.12922

5. Arent, Shawn M et al. "Nutrient Timing: A Garage Door of Opportunity?." Nutrients vol. 12,7 1948. 30 Jun. 2020, doi:10.3390/nu12071948

6. Mata, Fernando et al. "Carbohydrate Availability and Physical Performance: Physiological Overview and Practical Recommendations." Nutrients vol. 11,5 1084. 16 May. 2019, doi:10.3390/nu11051084

7. Escobar, Kurt A et al. "The Effect of a Moderately Low and High Carbohydrate Intake on Crossfit Performance." International journal of exercise science vol. 9,3 460-470. 1 Oct. 2016

8. Mata, Fernando et al. "Carbohydrate Availability and Physical Performance: Physiological Overview and Practical Recommendations." Nutrients vol. 11,5 1084. 16 May. 2019, doi:10.3390/nu11051084

I worked hard on this book, once you've finished reading, it would mean a lot to me if you could leave a review on Amazon. It would help spread the word about this material.

PART 2: RECIPES AND MEAL PLANS

Chapter 6: Shopping List

High-Carb Day

Complex Carbohydrates:

- Brown rice
- Quinoa
- Sweet potatoes
- Oats
- Whole-grain pasta
- Whole grain bread
- Rye bread

Fruits:

- Bananas
- Berries (strawberries, blueberries, raspberries)
- Apples
- Oranges

Proteins:

- Chicken breast
- Turkey breast
- Fish (salmon, tuna)
- Lean beef
- Pork shoulder, pork tenderloin

Vegetables:

- Broccoli
- Asparagus
- Spinach
- Bell peppers
- Kale

Legumes:

- Lentils
- Chickpeas
- Black beans

Healthy Fats:

- Avocado
- Olive oil
- Nuts (almonds, walnuts)

Dairy or Alternatives:

- Greek yogurt
- Cottage cheese
- Milk (or plant-based alternatives like almond or soy milk)

Low-Carb Day

Proteins:

- Eggs
- Chicken
- Turkey
- Fish (salmon, cod)
- Lean beef
- Pork tenderloin, pork loin

Vegetables:

- Leafy greens (spinach, kale, lettuce)
- Broccoli
- Cauliflower
- Zucchini
- Brussels sprouts

Healthy Fats:

- Avocado
- Olive oil
- Coconut oil

Dairy or Alternatives:

- Cheese (preferably low-fat)
- Greek yogurt (unsweetened)

Nuts and Seeds:

- Almonds
- Walnuts
- Chia seeds
- Flaxseeds

Beverages:

- Water
- Herbal teas
- Black coffee (unsweetened)

Condiments:

- Mustard
- Vinegar
- Herbs and spices (for flavor without added sugars)

Chapter 7: Low-Carb Recipes

Low-Carb Breakfast Recipes

Avocado and Bacon Egg Cups

Preparation time: 10 minutes

Cooking time: 15 minutes

Servings: 2

Ingredients:

- 2 avocados, halved and pitted
- 4 eggs
- 4 slices of bacon, cooked and crumbled
- Salt and pepper to taste
- Chopped chives for garnish (optional)

Directions:

1. Preheat the oven to 375°F.

2. Scoop out a small portion of each avocado half to create a well.

3. Place avocados in a baking dish to prevent tipping.

4. Crack an egg into each avocado half.

5. Sprinkle using crumbled bacon, salt, and pepper.

6. Bake for 15 minutes or 'til eggs are cooked to your liking.

7. Garnish using chopped chives if desired.

Per serving: Calories: 320kcal; Fat: 26g; Protein: 14g; Carbs: 9g; Sugar: 1g; Fiber: 7g

Spinach and Feta Omelet

Preparation time: 5 minutes

Cooking time: 7 minutes

Servings: 1

Ingredients:

- 2 large eggs
- 1 cup fresh spinach, chopped
- 2 tbsp feta cheese, crumbled
- Salt and pepper to taste
- Olive oil for cooking

Directions:

1. Whisk eggs in a bowl then season using salt and pepper.

2. Heat olive oil in a non-stick skillet in medium heat.

3. Add spinach to your skillet then sauté until wilted.

4. Pour whisked eggs over the spinach.

5. Sprinkle feta cheese over half of the omelet.

6. Cook 'til the eggs are set, then fold the omelet in half.

7. Serve hot.

Per serving: Calories: 280kcal; Fat: 20g; Protein: 18g; Carbs: 4g; Sugar: 1g; Fiber: 2g

Keto Chia Seed Pudding

Preparation time: 5 minutes (plus overnight chilling)

Cooking time: 0 minutes

Servings: 2

Ingredients:

- 1 cup unsweetened almond milk
- 2 tbsp chia seeds
- 1 tsp vanilla extract
- 1 tbsp low-carb sweetener (like stevia or erythritol)
- Berries for topping (optional)

Directions:

1. In your bowl, mix almond milk, chia seeds, vanilla extract, and sweetener.
2. Stir well then refrigerate overnight or for at least 4 hours.
3. Stir the mixture before serving.
4. Top with berries if desired.

Per serving: Calories: 120kcal; Fat: 9g; Protein: 4g; Carbs: 6g; Sugar: 1g; Fiber: 5g

Zucchini and Cheese Muffins

Preparation time: 10 minutes

Cooking time: 25 minutes

Servings: 6

Ingredients:

- 2 medium zucchinis, grated
- 4 eggs
- 1 cup shredded cheddar cheese
- 1/4 cup almond flour
- 1/2 tsp baking powder
- Salt and pepper to taste
- Chopped fresh herbs (optional)

Directions:

1. Preheat the oven to 375 deg. F then grease your muffin tin.
2. Squeeze excess moisture from grated zucchinis.
3. In your bowl, whisk together eggs, almond flour, baking powder, salt, and pepper.
4. Add grated zucchini and cheddar cheese to the egg mixture. Mix well.
5. Spoon the mixture into muffin cups and sprinkle with fresh herbs if desired.
6. Bake for 25 minutes or 'til muffins are set and golden.

Per serving: Calories: 150kcal; Fat: 11g; Protein: 9g; Carbs: 4g; Sugar: 2g; Fiber: 1g

Smoked Salmon and Cream Cheese Roll-Ups

Preparation time: 10 minutes

Cooking time: 0 minutes

Servings: 2

Ingredients:

- 4 oz smoked salmon slices
- 1/2 cup cream cheese
- 1 tbsp capers, drained
- Fresh dill for garnish

Directions:

1. Lay out smoked salmon slices on a clean surface.

2. Spread your thin layer of cream cheese on each slice.

3. Sprinkle capers evenly over the cream cheese.

4. Roll up the smoked salmon slices.

5. Garnish using fresh dill before serving.

Per serving: Calories: 280kcal; Fat: 22g; Protein: 18g; Carbs: 2g; Sugar: 1g; Fiber: 0g

Cauliflower Hash Browns

Preparation time: 15 minutes

Cooking time: 15 minutes

Servings: 4

Ingredients:

- 2 cups cauliflower rice
- 1/4 cup grated Parmesan cheese
- 1/4 cup almond flour
- 1 large egg
- 1/2 tsp garlic powder
- Salt and pepper to taste
- Olive oil for cooking

Directions:

1. In your bowl, combine salt, cauliflower rice, Parmesan cheese, almond flour, egg, garlic powder, and pepper.

2. Heat olive oil in your skillet in medium heat.

3. Spoon the cauliflower mixture onto your skillet to form small patties.

4. Cook 'til golden brown on both sides, about 7-8 minutes per side.

Per serving: Calories: 120kcal; Fat: 8g; Protein: 6g; Carbs: 6g; Sugar: 2g; Fiber: 2g

Keto Egg Salad Lettuce Wraps

Preparation time: 10 minutes

Cooking time: 0 minutes

Servings: 2

Ingredients:

- 4 hard-boiled eggs, chopped
- 1/4 cup mayonnaise
- 1 tsp Dijon mustard
- Salt and pepper to taste
- Lettuce leaves for wrapping

Directions:

1. In your bowl, combine chopped hard-boiled eggs, mayonnaise, Dijon mustard, salt, and pepper.
2. Mix well 'til all ingredients are evenly combined.
3. Spoon the egg salad onto lettuce leaves.
4. Wrap and secure with toothpicks if needed.

Per serving: Calories: 320kcal; Fat: 30g; Protein: 12g; Carbs: 2g; Sugar: 1g; Fiber: 1g

Almond Flour Pancakes

Preparation time: 10 minutes

Cooking time: 10 minutes

Servings: 2

Ingredients:

- 1 cup almond flour
- 2 eggs
- 1/2 cup unsweetened almond milk
- 1 tsp baking powder
- 1 tsp vanilla extract
- Butter or coconut oil for cooking

Directions:

1. In your bowl, whisk together almond flour, eggs, almond milk, baking powder, and vanilla extract.
2. Heat butter or coconut oil in your skillet in medium heat.
3. Spoon batter onto your skillet to form pancakes.
4. Cook 'til bubbles form on the surface, then flip then cook the other side.

Per serving: Calories: 450kcal; Fat: 38g; Protein: 18g; Carbs: 10g; Sugar: 2g; Fiber: 5g

Broccoli and Cheddar Breakfast Muffins

Preparation time: 15 minutes

Cooking time: 25 minutes

Servings: 6

Ingredients:

- 2 cups broccoli, finely chopped
- 4 large eggs
- 1 cup shredded cheddar cheese
- 1/4 cup almond flour
- 1/2 tsp baking powder
- Salt and pepper to taste

Directions:

1. Preheat the oven to 375 deg. F then grease your muffin tin.
2. In your bowl, whisk eggs and stir in broccoli, cheddar cheese, almond flour, baking powder, salt, and pepper.
3. Spoon the mixture into muffin cups.
4. Bake for 25 minutes or 'til muffins are set and slightly golden.

Per serving: Calories: 180kcal; Fat: 14g; Protein: 10g; Carbs: 4g; Sugar: 1g; Fiber: 2g

Turkey and Veggie Breakfast Skillet

Preparation time: 10 minutes

Cooking time: 15 minutes

Servings: 2

Ingredients:

- 1/2 lb ground turkey
- 1 bell pepper, diced
- 1 zucchini, diced
- 2 tbsp olive oil
- 1 tsp garlic powder
- Salt and pepper to taste
- 4 eggs

Directions:

1. In your skillet, heat olive oil in medium heat.
2. Add ground turkey, salt, garlic powder, and pepper. Cook 'til turkey is browned.
3. Add diced bell pepper and zucchini to your skillet. Cook 'til veggies are tender.
4. Make wells in the mixture then crack eggs into them.
5. Cover then cook 'til eggs are done to your liking.

Per serving: Calories: 380kcal; Fat: 28g; Protein: 24g; Carbs: 8g; Sugar: 4g; Fiber: 2g

Low-Carb Beef, Pork, and Poultry Recipes

Grilled Lemon Garlic Chicken

Preparation time: 10 minutes

Marinating time: 30 minutes

Cooking time: 15 minutes

Servings: 4

Ingredients:

- 4 boneless, skinless chicken breasts
- 1/4 cup olive oil
- Zest and juice of 1 lemon
- 3 cloves garlic, minced
- 1 tsp dried oregano
- Salt and pepper to taste

Directions:

1. In your bowl, mix olive oil, lemon zest, lemon juice, minced garlic, dried oregano, salt, and pepper.

2. Place chicken breasts in a resealable bag then pour the marinade over them. Marinate in the refrigerator for at least 30 minutes.

3. Preheat the grill to medium-high heat.

4. Grill the chicken for about 6-8 minutes per side or 'til fully cooked.

Per serving: Calories: 280kcal; Fat: 14g; Protein: 32g; Carbs: 2g; Sugar: 1g; Fiber: 0g

Beef and Vegetable Stir-Fry

Preparation time: 15 minutes

Cooking time: 10 minutes

Servings: 4

Ingredients:

- 1 lb beef sirloin, that is thinly sliced
- 2 cups broccoli florets
- 1 bell pepper, that is thinly sliced
- 1 cup snap peas
- 3 tbsp soy sauce
- 2 tbsp olive oil
- 1 tsp ginger, minced
- 2 cloves garlic, minced

Directions:

1. In your bowl, marinate beef slices with soy sauce, ginger, and garlic.

2. Heat olive oil in your wok or skillet over high heat.

3. Stir-fry beef until browned, then add vegetables and continue cooking until tender-crisp.

4. Serve hot.

Per serving: Calories: 320kcal; Fat: 18g; Protein: 28g; Carbs: 9g; Sugar: 3g; Fiber: 3g

Pork Tenderloin with Dijon Mustard Glaze

Preparation time: 10 minutes

Cooking time: 25 minutes

Servings: 4

Ingredients:

- 1 lb pork tenderloin
- 2 tbsp Dijon mustard
- 1 tbsp olive oil
- 1 tsp dried thyme
- Salt and pepper to taste

Directions:

1. Preheat the oven to 375°F.
2. Season pork tenderloin with salt, pepper, and dried thyme.
3. In your small bowl, mix Dijon mustard and olive oil. Brush the mixture over the pork.
4. Roast in to your oven for 25 minutes or 'til the internal temperature reaches 145°F.

Per serving: Calories: 250kcal; Fat: 12g; Protein: 32g; Carbs: 1g; Sugar: 0g; Fiber: 0g

Baked Turkey Meatballs with Zucchini

Preparation time: 15 minutes

Cooking time: 25 minutes

Servings: 4

Ingredients:

- 1 lb ground turkey
- 1/2 cup almond flour
- 1/4 cup grated Parmesan cheese
- 1 egg
- 1 tsp garlic powder
- 1/2 tsp dried oregano
- Salt and pepper to taste
- 1 zucchini, spiralized

Directions:

1. Preheat the oven to 400 deg. F then grease your baking sheet.
2. In your bowl, combine ground turkey, almond flour, Parmesan cheese, egg, garlic powder, oregano, salt, and pepper.
3. Form the mixture into meatballs and place them on your baking sheet.
4. Bake for 25 minutes or 'til the meatballs are cooked through.
5. Serve over spiralized zucchini.

Per serving: Calories: 280kcal; Fat: 18g; Protein: 24g; Carbs: 6g; Sugar: 2g; Fiber: 2g

Lemon Herb Grilled Steak

Preparation time: 10 minutes

Marinating time: 30 minutes

Cooking time: 10 minutes

Servings: 2

Ingredients:

- 2 beef steaks (such as sirloin or ribeye)
- Zest and juice of 1 lemon
- 2 tbsp olive oil
- 2 cloves garlic, minced
- 1 tsp dried thyme
- Salt and pepper to taste

Directions:

1. In your bowl, whisk together lemon zest, lemon juice, olive oil, minced garlic, dried thyme, salt, and pepper.

2. Marinate your steaks in the mixture for at least 30 minutes.

3. Preheat the grill to medium-high heat.

4. Grill the steaks for about 4-5 minutes per side or 'til they reach your desired doneness.

Per serving: Calories: 450kcal; Fat: 32g; Protein: 36g; Carbs: 2g; Sugar: 1g; Fiber: 0g

Cabbage and Beef Skillet

Preparation time: 10 minutes

Cooking time: 20 minutes

Servings: 4

Ingredients:

- 1 lb ground beef
- 1 small cabbage, shredded
- 1 onion, diced
- 2 cloves garlic, minced
- 1 tsp cumin
- 1 tsp paprika
- Salt and pepper to taste
- Olive oil for cooking

Directions:

1. In your large skillet, heat olive oil in medium heat.

2. Add ground beef, onion, and garlic. Cook 'til beef is browned.

3. Add shredded cabbage, cumin, paprika, salt, and pepper. Cook 'til cabbage is tender.

4. Serve hot.

Per serving: Calories: 380kcal; Fat: 28g; Protein: 24g; Carbs: 10g; Sugar: 6g; Fiber: 4g

Rosemary Roasted Pork Loin

Preparation time: 10 minutes

Cooking time: 45 minutes

Servings: 4

Ingredients:

- 1 lb pork loin
- 2 tbsp olive oil
- 2 tsp dried rosemary
- 1 tsp garlic powder
- Salt and pepper to taste

Directions:

1. Preheat the oven to 400°F.
2. Rub pork loin with olive oil, dried rosemary, garlic powder, salt, and pepper.
3. Place the pork loin in your roasting pan.
4. Roast in to your oven for 45 minutes or 'til the internal temperature reaches 145°F.

Per serving: Calories: 320kcal; Fat: 20g; Protein: 32g; Carbs: 0g; Sugar: 0g; Fiber: 0g

Chicken and Broccoli Casserole

Preparation time: 15 minutes

Cooking time: 30 minutes

Servings: 4

Ingredients:

- 1 lb boneless, skinless chicken breasts, that is cooked and shredded
- 2 cups broccoli florets, steamed
- 1 cup shredded cheddar cheese
- 1/2 cup mayonnaise
- 1/2 cup sour cream
- 1 tsp garlic powder
- Salt and pepper to taste

Directions:

1. Preheat the oven to 350°F.
2. In your bowl, mix shredded chicken, steamed broccoli, cheddar cheese, mayonnaise, sour cream, garlic powder, salt, and pepper.
3. Transfer the mixture to a baking dish.
4. Bake for 30 minutes or 'til the top is golden and bubbly.

Per serving: Calories: 420kcal; Fat: 32g; Protein: 24g; Carbs: 6g; Sugar: 2g; Fiber: 2g

Spicy Ground Turkey Lettuce Wraps

Preparation time: 15 minutes

Cooking time: 15 minutes

Servings: 4

Ingredients:

- 1 lb ground turkey
- 1 tbsp olive oil
- 1 onion, diced
- 2 cloves garlic, minced
- 1 tsp ground cumin
- 1 tsp chili powder
- 1/2 tsp cayenne pepper (adjust to taste)
- Salt and pepper to taste
- Iceberg lettuce leaves for wrapping

Directions:

1. In your skillet, heat olive oil in medium heat.
2. Add diced onion and minced garlic. Cook 'til softened.
3. Add ground turkey then cook 'til browned.
4. Stir in cumin, chili powder, cayenne pepper, salt, and pepper.
5. Spoon your mixture into lettuce leaves for wrapping.

Per serving: Calories: 240kcal; Fat: 15g; Protein: 20g; Carbs: 7g; Sugar: 2g; Fiber: 2g

Crispy Baked Chicken Thighs

Preparation time: 10 minutes

Cooking time: 35 minutes

Servings: 4

Ingredients:

- 4 chicken thighs, bone-in, skin-on
- 2 tbsp olive oil
- 1 tsp paprika
- 1 tsp garlic powder
- 1/2 tsp dried thyme
- Salt and pepper to taste

Directions:

1. Preheat the oven to 425 deg. F then line your baking sheet using parchment paper.
2. Pat chicken thighs dry using paper towels.
3. Rub chicken thighs with olive oil, paprika, garlic powder, dried thyme, salt, and pepper.
4. Place the chicken thighs on your prepared baking sheet then bake for 35 minutes or 'til the skin is crispy.

Per serving: Calories: 320kcal; Fat: 25g; Protein: 20g; Carbs: 1g; Sugar: 0g; Fiber: 0g

Italian Sausage and Peppers

Preparation time: 10 minutes

Cooking time: 25 minutes

Servings: 4

Ingredients:

- 1 lb Italian sausage links
- 2 bell peppers, sliced
- 1 onion, sliced
- 2 cloves garlic, minced
- 1 can (14 oz) diced tomatoes
- 1 tsp dried oregano
- 1 tsp dried basil
- Salt and pepper to taste

Directions:

1. In your skillet, brown the Italian sausage in medium heat.
2. Add sliced bell peppers, sliced onions, and minced garlic. Cook 'til vegetables are tender.
3. Stir in diced tomatoes, oregano, basil, salt, and pepper. Simmer for 10 minutes.
4. Serve hot.

Per serving: Calories: 480kcal; Fat: 36g; Protein: 20g; Carbs: 12g; Sugar: 6g; Fiber: 3g

Low-Carb Fish and Seafood Recipes

Lemon Garlic Butter Baked Salmon

Preparation time: 10 minutes

Cooking time: 15 minutes

Servings: 4

Ingredients:

- 4 salmon fillets
- 4 tbsp unsalted butter, melted
- 3 cloves garlic, minced
- Zest and juice of 1 lemon
- 1 tsp dried dill
- Salt and pepper to taste

Directions:

1. Preheat the oven to 400 deg. F then line your baking sheet using parchment paper.
2. Place salmon fillets on your baking sheet.
3. In your bowl, mix melted butter, minced garlic, lemon zest, lemon juice, dried dill, salt, and pepper.
4. Brush the butter mixture over the salmon.
5. Bake for 15 minutes or 'til the salmon is cooked through.

Per serving: Calories: 350kcal; Fat: 25g; Protein: 30g; Carbs: 1g; Sugar: 0g; Fiber: 0g

Shrimp and Avocado Salad

Preparation time: 15 minutes

Cooking time: 0 minutes

Servings: 2

Ingredients:

- 1 lb shrimp, cooked and peeled
- 2 avocados, diced
- 1 cup cherry tomatoes, halved
- 1/4 cup red onion, finely chopped
- 2 tbsp olive oil
- 1 tbsp fresh cilantro, chopped
- Zest and juice of 1 lime
- Salt and pepper to taste

Directions:

1. In your bowl, combine shrimp, diced avocados, cherry tomatoes, and chopped red onion.

2. In your separate bowl, whisk together olive oil, chopped cilantro, lime zest, lime juice, salt, and pepper.

3. Place dressing over the shrimp mixture then toss gently.

4. Serve chilled.

Per serving: Calories: 420kcal; Fat: 28g; Protein: 32g; Carbs: 18g; Sugar: 4g; Fiber: 12g

Baked Cod with Herbs and Lemon

Preparation time: 10 minutes

Cooking time: 15 minutes

Servings: 4

Ingredients:

- 4 cod fillets
- 2 tbsp olive oil
- 1 tsp dried thyme
- 1 tsp dried rosemary
- Zest and juice of 1 lemon
- Salt and pepper to taste

Directions:

1. Preheat the oven to 400 deg. F then line your baking sheet using parchment paper.

2. Place cod fillets on your baking sheet.

3. In your bowl, mix olive oil, dried thyme, dried rosemary, lemon zest, lemon juice, salt, and pepper.

4. Brush herb mixture over the cod fillets.

5. Bake for 15 minutes or 'til the cod is flaky.

Per serving: Calories: 220kcal; Fat: 10g; Protein: 30g; Carbs: 2g; Sugar: 0g; Fiber: 1g

Tuna Salad Lettuce Wraps

Preparation time: 10 minutes

Cooking time: 0 minutes

Servings: 2

Ingredients:

- 2 cans (5 oz each) tuna, drained
- 1/4 cup mayonnaise
- 1 celery stalk, finely chopped
- 2 tbsp red onion, finely chopped
- 1 tbsp Dijon mustard
- Salt and pepper to taste
- Lettuce leaves for wrapping

Directions:

1. In your bowl, combine drained tuna, mayonnaise, chopped celery, chopped red onion, Dijon mustard, salt, and pepper.

2. Mix well 'til all ingredients are evenly combined.

3. Spoon the tuna salad into lettuce leaves for wrapping.

4. Serve chilled.

Per serving: Calories: 320kcal; Fat: 25g; Protein: 20g; Carbs: 4g; Sugar: 1g; Fiber: 1g

Grilled Garlic Butter Shrimp Skewers

Preparation time: 15 minutes

Cooking time: 5 minutes

Servings: 4

Ingredients:

- 1 lb large shrimp, peeled and deveined
- 1/4 cup unsalted butter, melted
- 3 cloves garlic, minced
- 1 tbsp fresh parsley, chopped
- Zest and juice of 1 lemon
- Salt and pepper to taste
- Skewers, soaked in water

Directions:

1. Preheat the grill to medium-high heat.

2. In your bowl, mix melted butter, minced garlic, chopped parsley, lemon zest, lemon juice, salt, and pepper.

3. Thread shrimp onto skewers then brush with the garlic butter mixture.

4. Grill for 2-3 minutes per side or 'til shrimp are opaque then cooked through.

Per serving: Calories: 220kcal; Fat: 15g; Protein: 18g; Carbs: 2g; Sugar: 0g; Fiber: 0g

Fish Taco Lettuce Wraps

Preparation time: 15 minutes

Cooking time: 10 minutes

Servings: 4

Ingredients:

- 1 lb white fish fillets (e.g., cod or tilapia)
- 1 tbsp olive oil
- 1 tsp chili powder
- 1/2 tsp cumin
- 1/2 tsp paprika
- Salt and pepper to taste
- Iceberg lettuce leaves for wrapping
- Sliced avocado, salsa, and cilantro for topping

Directions:

1. Season fish fillets with olive oil, chili powder, cumin, paprika, salt, and pepper.

2. Heat your skillet in medium heat then cook the fish for 4-5 minutes per side or 'til flaky.

3. Break fish into smaller pieces and place them in lettuce leaves.

4. Top with sliced avocado, salsa, and cilantro.

Per serving: Calories: 180kcal; Fat: 8g; Protein: 22g; Carbs: 6g; Sugar: 2g; Fiber: 3g

Spicy Cilantro Lime Tilapia

Preparation time: 10 minutes

Cooking time: 10 minutes

Servings: 4

Ingredients:

- 4 tilapia fillets
- 2 tbsp olive oil
- 2 tbsp fresh cilantro, chopped
- Zest and juice of 2 limes
- 1 tsp chili powder
- 1/2 tsp cayenne pepper (adjust to taste)
- Salt and pepper to taste

Directions:

1. In your bowl, mix olive oil, chopped cilantro, lime zest, lime juice, chili powder, cayenne pepper, salt, and pepper.

2. Rub the tilapia fillets with the mixture.

3. Heat your skillet in medium heat then cook the tilapia for 4-5 minutes per side or 'til it flakes easily.

Per serving: Calories: 180kcal; Fat: 10g; Protein: 22g; Carbs: 2g; Sugar: 0g; Fiber: 0g

Zucchini Noodles with Pesto and Shrimp

Preparation time: 15 minutes

Cooking time: 10 minutes

Servings: 2

Ingredients:

- 2 medium zucchinis, spiralized
- 1 lb large shrimp, peeled and deveined
- 1/4 cup pesto sauce
- 1 tbsp olive oil
- Cherry tomatoes for garnish
- Parmesan cheese for topping (optional)

Directions:

1. In your skillet, heat olive oil in medium heat.
2. Add shrimp then cook for 2-3 minutes per side or 'til opaque.
3. Add zucchini noodles to your skillet then toss with pesto until heated through.
4. Serve with cherry tomatoes and top with Parmesan cheese if desired.

Per serving: Calories: 320kcal; Fat: 20g; Protein: 28g; Carbs: 10g; Sugar: 6g; Fiber: 4g

Keto Crab Cakes

Preparation time: 15 minutes

Cooking time: 10 minutes

Servings: 4

Ingredients:

- 1 lb lump crabmeat, drained
- 1/4 cup almond flour
- 2 tbsp mayonnaise
- 1 egg
- 1 tsp Dijon mustard
- 1 tbsp fresh parsley, chopped
- 1/2 tsp Old Bay seasoning
- Salt and pepper to taste
- 2 tbsp olive oil for cooking

Directions:

1. In your bowl, combine crabmeat, almond flour, mayonnaise, egg, Dijon mustard, chopped parsley, Old Bay seasoning, salt, and pepper.
2. Form the mixture into crab cakes.
3. Heat olive oil in your skillet in medium heat.
4. Cook crab cakes for 3-4 minutes per side or 'til golden brown.

Per serving: Calories: 180kcal; Fat: 12g; Protein: 15g; Carbs: 2g; Sugar: 0g; Fiber: 1g

Garlic Butter Scallops

Preparation time: 10 minutes

Cooking time: 5 minutes

Servings: 2

Ingredients:

- 1 lb scallops
- 3 tbsp unsalted butter
- 3 cloves garlic, minced
- 1 tbsp fresh parsley, chopped
- Salt and pepper to taste
- Lemon wedges for serving

Directions:

1. Pat the scallops dry using paper towels then season using salt and pepper.

2. In your skillet, melt butter in medium-high heat.

3. Add minced garlic then sauté for 1-2 minutes.

4. Add scallops to your skillet then cook for 2-3 minutes per side or 'til they are opaque.

5. Sprinkle using chopped parsley then serve with lemon wedges.

Per serving: Calories: 280kcal; Fat: 20g; Protein: 25g; Carbs: 4g; Sugar: 0g; Fiber: 0g

Smoked Salmon Cucumber Bites

Preparation time: 10 minutes

Cooking time: 0 minutes

Servings: 4

Ingredients:

- 1 cucumber, sliced
- 4 oz smoked salmon
- 1/4 cup cream cheese
- Fresh dill for garnish

Directions:

1. Place cucumber slices on your serving platter.

2. Top each cucumber slice with a small amount of cream cheese.

3. Add a piece of your smoked salmon on top.

4. Garnish using fresh dill.

Per serving: Calories: 120kcal; Fat: 8g; Protein: 8g; Carbs: 3g; Sugar: 1g; Fiber: 1g

Coconut Lime Grilled Mahi-Mahi

Preparation time: 15 minutes

Cooking time: 10 minutes

Servings: 2

Ingredients:

- 2 mahi-mahi fillets
- 2 tbsp coconut oil, melted
- Zest and juice of 1 lime
- 1 tsp chili powder
- 1/2 tsp ground cumin
- Salt and pepper to taste
- Fresh cilantro for garnish

Directions:

1. In your bowl, whisk together melted coconut oil, lime zest, lime juice, chili powder, ground cumin, salt, and pepper.

2. Marinate mahi-mahi fillets in the mixture for at least 30 minutes.

3. Preheat the grill to medium-high heat.

4. Grill the mahi-mahi for 4-5 minutes per side or 'til it flakes easily.

5. Garnish using fresh cilantro before serving.

Per serving: Calories: 300kcal; Fat: 20g; Protein: 30g; Carbs: 2g; Sugar: 0g; Fiber: 0g

Low-Carb Rice, Pasta, and Soup Recipes

Cauliflower Fried Rice

Preparation time: 15 minutes

Cooking time: 10 minutes

Servings: 4

Ingredients:

- 1 head cauliflower, grated
- 2 tbsp sesame oil
- 1 cup mixed vegetables (peas, carrots, corn)
- 2 eggs, beaten
- 3 tbsp soy sauce
- 2 green onions, chopped
- Salt and pepper to taste

Directions:

1. In your large skillet, heat sesame oil in medium heat.

2. Add grated cauliflower and mixed vegetables. Stir-fry for 5-7 minutes 'til vegetables are tender.

3. Push the cauliflower mixture to the side of the skillet then pour beaten eggs into the empty side.

4. Scramble the eggs and mix them with the cauliflower.

5. Stir in soy sauce, green onions, salt, and pepper. Cook for an additional 2-3 minutes.

Per serving: Calories: 150kcal; Fat: 9g; Protein: 7g; Carbs: 12g; Sugar: 5g; Fiber: 5g

Broccoli and Cheese Soup

Preparation time: 10 minutes

Cooking time: 20 minutes

Servings: 4

Ingredients:

- 4 cups broccoli florets
- 2 cups cauliflower florets
- 1/4 cup unsalted butter
- 1/4 cup almond flour
- 4 cups vegetable broth
- 2 cups shredded cheddar cheese
- 1 cup heavy cream
- Salt and pepper to taste

Directions:

1. In your pot, steam broccoli and cauliflower until tender.

2. In another pot, melt butter in medium heat. Stir in almond flour to make a roux.

3. Gradually whisk in vegetable broth 'til smooth.

4. Add steamed broccoli and cauliflower to the pot.

5. Stir in shredded cheddar cheese and heavy cream 'til the cheese is melted.

6. Season using salt and pepper. Simmer for 10 minutes.

Per serving: Calories: 420kcal; Fat: 36g; Protein: 15g; Carbs: 10g; Sugar: 4g; Fiber: 4g

Shirataki Noodles with Alfredo Sauce

Preparation time: 10 minutes

Cooking time: 5 minutes

Servings: 2

Ingredients:

- 2 packs shirataki noodles, that is drained and rinsed
- 1/2 cup heavy cream
- 1/4 cup grated Parmesan cheese
- 2 tbsp unsalted butter
- 2 cloves garlic, minced
- Salt and pepper to taste
- Chopped parsley for garnish

Directions:

1. Rinse shirataki noodles under cold water and pat them dry.

2. In your skillet, melt butter in medium heat. Add minced garlic then sauté for 1 minute.

3. Pour in heavy cream then simmer.

4. Stir in Parmesan cheese 'til the sauce thickens.

5. Add shirataki noodles to your skillet then toss to coat.

6. Season using salt and pepper, garnish with chopped parsley, then serve.

Per serving: Calories: 320kcal; Fat: 28g; Protein: 6g; Carbs: 8g; Sugar: 2g; Fiber: 3g

Mexican Cauliflower Rice

Preparation time: 15 minutes

Cooking time: 10 minutes

Servings: 4

Ingredients:

- 1 head cauliflower, grated
- 1 tbsp olive oil
- 1/2 onion, diced
- 2 cloves garlic, minced
- 1 cup diced tomatoes
- 1/2 cup bell peppers, diced
- 1 tsp ground cumin
- 1 tsp chili powder
- Salt and pepper to taste
- Fresh cilantro for garnish

Directions:

1. In your large skillet, heat olive oil in medium heat.

2. Add diced onion and minced garlic. Sauté 'til softened.

3. Stir in grated cauliflower, diced tomatoes, and bell peppers.

4. Season using ground cumin, chili powder, salt, and pepper. Cook for 5-7 minutes.

5. Garnish using fresh cilantro before serving.

Per serving: Calories: 90kcal; Fat: 4g; Protein: 3g; Carbs: 12g; Sugar: 5g; Fiber: 5g

Spinach and Sausage Soup

Preparation time: 15 minutes

Cooking time: 25 minutes

Servings: 4

Ingredients:

- 1 lb Italian sausage, casings removed
- 1 onion, diced
- 2 cloves garlic, minced
- 4 cups chicken broth
- 1 can (14 oz) diced tomatoes
- 1 tsp dried oregano
- 1 tsp dried basil
- Salt and pepper to taste
- 4 cups fresh spinach
- Parmesan cheese for garnish

Directions:

1. In your large pot, cook Italian sausage in medium heat, breaking it into crumbles.

2. Add diced onion and minced garlic. Cook 'til sausage is browned and onions are translucent.

3. Stir in chicken broth, diced tomatoes, oregano, basil, salt, and pepper. Bring to a simmer.

4. Add fresh spinach then cook 'til wilted.

5. Serve hot, garnished with Parmesan cheese.

Per serving: Calories: 320kcal; Fat: 22g; Protein: 16g; Carbs: 15g; Sugar: 6g; Fiber: 5g

Egg Drop Soup

Preparation time: 5 minutes

Cooking time: 10 minutes

Servings: 2

Ingredients:

- 4 cups chicken broth
- 2 eggs, beaten
- 2 green onions, sliced
- 1 tsp soy sauce
- 1/2 tsp sesame oil
- Salt and pepper to taste

Directions:

1. In your pot, bring chicken broth to a simmer.

2. Slowly pour beaten eggs into the simmering broth, stirring continuously.

3. Add sliced green onions, soy sauce, sesame oil, salt, and pepper.

4. Continue to stir 'til the eggs are cooked and soup is heated through.

Per serving: Calories: 100kcal; Fat: 6g; Protein: 8g; Carbs: 4g; Sugar: 0g; Fiber: 1g

Creamy Tomato Basil Zoodle Soup

Preparation time: 10 minutes

Cooking time: 15 minutes

Servings: 4

Ingredients:

- 4 cups vegetable broth
- 1 can (14 oz) crushed tomatoes
- 2 cloves garlic, minced
- 1 tsp dried basil
- 1/2 cup heavy cream
- 4 zucchinis, spiralized
- Salt and pepper to taste
- Fresh basil for garnish

Directions:

1. In your pot, combine vegetable broth, crushed tomatoes, minced garlic, and dried basil. Bring to a simmer.

2. Stir in heavy cream and add spiralized zucchini. Cook for 5-7 minutes until zoodles are tender.

3. Season using salt and pepper.

4. Garnish using fresh basil before serving.

Per serving: Calories: 180kcal; Fat: 15g; Protein: 3g; Carbs: 10g; Sugar: 6g; Fiber: 3g

Spaghetti Squash with Meat Sauce

Preparation time: 15 minutes

Cooking time: 50 minutes

Servings: 4

Ingredients:

- 1 spaghetti squash, that is halved and seeds removed
- 1 lb ground beef
- 1/2 onion, diced
- 2 cloves garlic, minced
- 1 can (14 oz) crushed tomatoes
- 1 tsp dried oregano
- 1 tsp dried basil
- Salt and pepper to taste
- Fresh parsley for garnish
- Parmesan cheese for topping (optional)

Directions:

1. Preheat the oven to 375°F.

2. Place spaghetti squash halves, cut side down, on your baking sheet. Bake for 40-45 minutes or 'til tender.

3. In your skillet, cook ground beef in medium heat until browned. Add diced onion and minced garlic, cooking 'til softened.

4. Stir in crushed tomatoes, dried oregano, dried basil, salt, and pepper. Simmer for 10 minutes.

5. Scrape the spaghetti squash using a fork to create "noodles." Top with meat sauce, garnish with fresh parsley, and optionally sprinkle with Parmesan cheese.

Per serving: Calories: 300kcal; Fat: 15g; Protein: 20g; Carbs: 25g; Sugar: 10g; Fiber: 5g

Creamy Cauliflower and Bacon Soup

Preparation time: 15 minutes

Cooking time: 25 minutes

Servings: 4

Ingredients:

- 1 head cauliflower, chopped
- 4 cups chicken broth
- 6 slices bacon, cooked and crumbled
- 1/2 onion, diced
- 2 cloves garlic, minced
- 1/2 cup heavy cream
- Salt and pepper to taste
- Chives for garnish

Directions:

1. In your large pot, combine chopped cauliflower and chicken broth. Bring to a boil then simmer 'til cauliflower is tender.

2. Meanwhile, cook bacon until crispy. Set aside.

3. In your skillet, sauté diced onion and minced garlic 'til softened.

4. Place onion and garlic mixture to the pot of cauliflower. Use immersion blender to puree 'til smooth.

5. Stir in heavy cream, crumbled bacon, salt, and pepper. Simmer for an additional 5 minutes.

6. Garnish using chives before serving.

Per serving: Calories: 280kcal; Fat: 22g; Protein: 8g; Carbs: 14g; Sugar: 5g; Fiber: 5g

Low-Carb Chicken and Vegetable Stir-Fry

Preparation time: 15 minutes

Cooking time: 15 minutes

Servings: 4

Ingredients:

- 1 lb boneless, skinless chicken breasts, that is thinly sliced
- 2 tbsp soy sauce
- 1 tbsp olive oil
- 1 bell pepper, that is thinly sliced
- 1 zucchini, that is thinly sliced
- 1 cup broccoli florets
- 2 cloves garlic, minced
- 1 tsp ginger, grated
- Salt and pepper to taste
- Sesame seeds for garnish

Directions:

1. In your bowl, marinate chicken slices in soy sauce.
2. Heat olive oil in your wok or skillet over high heat.
3. Add marinated chicken and stir-fry until browned then cooked through.
4. Add sliced bell pepper, zucchini, broccoli, minced garlic, and grated ginger. Stir-fry for an additional 5-7 minutes 'til vegetables are tender.
5. Season using salt and pepper. Garnish using sesame seeds before serving.

Per serving: Calories: 220kcal; Fat: 10g; Protein: 25g; Carbs: 8g; Sugar: 4g; Fiber: 3g

Low-Carb Vegetarian Recipes

Caprese Salad with Balsamic Glaze

Preparation time: 10 minutes

Cooking time: 0 minutes

Servings: 2

Ingredients:

- 2 large tomatoes, sliced
- 1 ball fresh mozzarella, sliced
- Fresh basil leaves
- 2 tbsp extra virgin olive oil
- 1 tbsp balsamic glaze
- Salt and pepper to taste

Directions:

1. Arrange tomato and mozzarella slices on your serving platter, alternating with basil leaves.
2. Drizzle using extra virgin olive oil and balsamic glaze.
3. Season using salt and pepper.
4. Serve immediately.

Per serving: Calories: 300kcal; Fat: 25g; Protein: 15g; Carbs: 8g; Sugar: 5g; Fiber: 2g

Cauliflower and Broccoli Gratin

Preparation time: 15 minutes

Cooking time: 25 minutes

Servings: 4

Ingredients:

- 1 head cauliflower, cut into florets
- 1 bunch broccoli, cut into florets
- 2 tbsp butter
- 2 tbsp almond flour
- 1 cup heavy cream
- 1 cup shredded cheddar cheese
- Salt and pepper to taste
- Chopped parsley for garnish

Directions:

1. Preheat the oven to 375°F.
2. Steam cauliflower and broccoli until slightly tender.
3. In your saucepan, melt butter and stir in almond flour to make a roux.
4. Gradually whisk in heavy cream 'til smooth.
5. Stir in shredded cheddar cheese until melted.
6. Combine the cheese sauce with steamed cauliflower and broccoli.
7. Transfer to a baking dish then bake for 25 minutes or 'til bubbly and golden.
8. Garnish using chopped parsley before serving.

Per serving: Calories: 350kcal; Fat: 28g; Protein: 12g; Carbs: 12g; Sugar: 4g; Fiber: 4g

Stuffed Bell Peppers with Cauliflower Rice

Preparation time: 20 minutes

Cooking time: 30 minutes

Servings: 4

Ingredients:

- 4 bell peppers, that is halved and seeds removed
- 2 cups cauliflower rice
- 1 cup black beans, that is drained and rinsed
- 1 cup cherry tomatoes, halved
- 1/2 cup red onion, finely chopped
- 1 cup shredded Monterey Jack cheese
- 1 tsp ground cumin
- 1 tsp chili powder
- Salt and pepper to taste
- Fresh cilantro for garnish

Directions:

1. Preheat the oven to 375°F.
2. In your bowl, mix cauliflower rice, black beans, cherry tomatoes, red onion, shredded cheese, ground cumin, chili powder, salt, and pepper.
3. Stuff the bell pepper halves with the cauliflower rice mixture.
4. Place stuffed peppers in a baking dish then bake for 30 minutes or 'til the peppers are tender.
5. Garnish using fresh cilantro before serving.

Per serving: Calories: 250kcal; Fat: 14g; Protein: 12g; Carbs: 20g; Sugar: 6g; Fiber: 6g

Creamy Avocado and Cucumber Salad

Preparation time: 10 minutes

Cooking time: 0 minutes

Servings: 2

Ingredients:

- 2 avocados, diced
- 1 cucumber, diced
- 1/4 red onion, finely chopped
- 2 tbsp sour cream
- 1 tbsp lime juice
- 1 tbsp fresh cilantro, chopped
- Salt and pepper to taste

Directions:

1. In your bowl, combine diced avocados, diced cucumber, and finely chopped red onion.

2. In your separate small bowl, whisk together sour cream, lime juice, chopped cilantro, salt, and pepper.

3. Place dressing over the avocado and cucumber mixture. Toss gently to coat.

4. Serve chilled.

Per serving: Calories: 320kcal; Fat: 28g; Protein: 4g; Carbs: 18g; Sugar: 4g; Fiber: 9g

Zucchini and Tomato Bake

Preparation time: 15 minutes

Cooking time: 25 minutes

Servings: 4

Ingredients:

- 2 zucchinis, sliced
- 2 tomatoes, sliced
- 1/4 cup grated Parmesan cheese
- 2 tbsp olive oil
- 1 tsp dried oregano
- 1 tsp dried basil
- Salt and pepper to taste
- Fresh parsley for garnish

Directions:

1. Preheat the oven to 375°F.

2. Arrange zucchini and tomato slices in a baking dish, alternating and overlapping.

3. Drizzle using olive oil and sprinkle with grated Parmesan, dried oregano, dried basil, salt, and pepper.

4. Bake for 25 minutes or 'til the vegetables are tender.

5. Garnish using fresh parsley before serving.

Per serving: Calories: 120kcal; Fat: 9g; Protein: 3g; Carbs: 8g; Sugar: 4g; Fiber: 3g

Keto Portobello Mushroom Pizzas

Preparation time: 10 minutes

Cooking time: 15 minutes

Servings: 2

Ingredients:

- 4 large portobello mushrooms, stems removed
- 1/2 cup sugar-free marinara sauce
- 1 cup shredded mozzarella cheese
- 1/4 cup sliced olives
- 1 tsp dried oregano
- Salt and pepper to taste
- Fresh basil for garnish

Directions:

1. Preheat the oven to 400°F.
2. Place portobello mushrooms on your baking sheet.
3. Spread marinara sauce over each mushroom cap.
4. Top with shredded mozzarella, sliced olives, dried oregano, salt, and pepper.
5. Bake for 15 minutes or 'til the cheese is melted and bubbly.
6. Garnish using fresh basil before serving.

Per serving: Calories: 270kcal; Fat: 18g; Protein: 17g; Carbs: 11g; Sugar: 5g; Fiber: 4g

Greek Salad with Tofu Feta

Preparation time: 15 minutes

Cooking time: 0 minutes

Servings: 4

Ingredients:

- 1 cucumber, diced
- 1 cup cherry tomatoes, halved
- 1/2 red onion, that is thinly sliced
- 1/2 cup Kalamata olives, pitted
- 1/2 cup crumbled tofu feta
- 2 tbsp olive oil
- 1 tbsp red wine vinegar
- 1 tsp dried oregano
- Salt and pepper to taste

Directions:

1. In your large bowl, combine diced cucumber, cherry tomatoes, that is thinly sliced red onion, Kalamata olives, and crumbled tofu feta.
2. In your small bowl, whisk together salt, olive oil, red wine vinegar, dried oregano, and pepper.
3. Place dressing over the salad then toss gently to combine.
4. Serve chilled.

Per serving: Calories: 220kcal; Fat: 18g; Protein: 8g; Carbs: 10g; Sugar: 5g; Fiber: 3g

Cabbage and Mushroom Skewers

Preparation time: 15 minutes

Cooking time: 10 minutes

Servings: 4

Ingredients:

- 1 small cabbage, cut into wedges
- 8 oz mushrooms, cleaned
- 2 tbsp olive oil
- 1 tsp smoked paprika
- 1 tsp garlic powder
- 1 tsp onion powder
- Salt and pepper to taste
- Wooden skewers, soaked in water

Directions:

1. Preheat the grill to medium-high heat.

2. Thread cabbage wedges and mushrooms onto soaked wooden skewers.

3. In your bowl, mix olive oil, smoked paprika, garlic powder, onion powder, salt, and pepper.

4. Brush the skewers using the olive oil mixture.

5. Grill for 5 minutes per side or 'til the vegetables are charred and tender.

Per serving: Calories: 120kcal; Fat: 8g; Protein: 3g; Carbs: 12g; Sugar: 6g; Fiber: 4g

Spaghetti Squash Primavera

Preparation time: 15 minutes

Cooking time: 40 minutes

Servings: 4

Ingredients:

- 1 large spaghetti squash, that is halved and seeds removed
- 2 tbsp olive oil
- 1 bell pepper, that is thinly sliced
- 1 zucchini, julienned
- 1 carrot, julienned
- 1 cup cherry tomatoes, halved
- 2 cloves garlic, minced
- 1/2 cup grated Parmesan cheese
- 1/4 cup fresh basil, chopped
- Salt and pepper to taste

Directions:

1. Preheat the oven to 375°F.

2. Place spaghetti squash halves, cut side down, on your baking sheet. Bake for 30-40 minutes or 'til tender.

3. In your large skillet, heat olive oil in medium heat. Add bell pepper, zucchini, carrot, and minced garlic. Sauté for 5-7 minutes 'til vegetables are tender.

4. Scrape the spaghetti squash using a fork to create "noodles" and add them to your skillet.

5. Stir in cherry tomatoes, grated Parmesan, and chopped basil. Cook for an additional 2-3 minutes.

6. Season using salt and pepper. Serve hot.

Per serving: Calories: 220kcal; Fat: 14g; Protein: 7g; Carbs: 20g; Sugar: 8g; Fiber: 5g

Avocado and Pecan Salad

Preparation time: 10 minutes

Cooking time: 0 minutes

Servings: 2

Ingredients:

- 2 avocados, diced
- 1 cup mixed salad greens
- 1/2 cup cherry tomatoes, halved
- 1/4 cup pecans, chopped
- 2 tbsp feta cheese, crumbled
- 2 tbsp balsamic vinaigrette dressing
- Salt and pepper to taste

Directions:

1. In your bowl, combine diced avocados, mixed salad greens, cherry tomatoes, chopped pecans, and crumbled feta cheese.

2. Drizzle using balsamic vinaigrette dressing.

3. Toss gently to combine then season using salt and pepper.

4. Serve immediately.

Per serving: Calories: 350kcal; Fat: 30g; Protein: 5g; Carbs: 20g; Sugar: 5g; Fiber: 10g

Cucumber and Avocado Salad

Preparation time: 10 minutes

Cooking time: 0 minutes

Servings: 2

Ingredients:

- 1 cucumber, that is thinly sliced
- 1 avocado, diced
- 1/4 red onion, that is thinly sliced
- 2 tbsp olive oil
- 1 tbsp fresh lemon juice
- 1 tbsp fresh cilantro, chopped
- Salt and pepper to taste

Directions:

1. In your bowl, combine cucumber slices, diced avocado, and thinly sliced red onion.

2. In your separate small bowl, whisk together olive oil, lemon juice, chopped cilantro, salt, and pepper.

3. Place dressing over the cucumber and avocado mixture. Toss gently to coat.

4. Serve chilled.

Per serving: Calories: 250kcal; Fat: 22g; Protein: 3g; Carbs: 14g; Sugar: 3g; Fiber: 7g

Creamy Asparagus and Spinach Soup

Preparation time: 10 minutes

Cooking time: 20 minutes

Servings: 4

Ingredients:

- 1 lb asparagus, trimmed and chopped
- 1 onion, diced
- 2 cloves garlic, minced
- 4 cups vegetable broth
- 2 cups fresh spinach
- 1/2 cup heavy cream
- 2 tbsp olive oil
- Salt and pepper to taste
- Lemon zest for garnish

Directions:

1. In your pot, heat olive oil in medium heat. Sauté diced onion and minced garlic 'til softened.

2. Add chopped asparagus then cook for 5 minutes.

3. Pour in vegetable broth then simmer. Cook for an additional 10-12 minutes until asparagus is tender.

4. Stir in fresh spinach then cook 'til wilted.

5. Use immersion blender to puree the soup 'til smooth.

6. Stir in heavy cream, season using salt and pepper, then simmer for 5 minutes.

7. Garnish using lemon zest before serving.

Per serving: Calories: 180kcal; Fat: 15g; Protein: 4g; Carbs: 10g; Sugar: 4g; Fiber: 4g

Broccoli and Cheese Stuffed Bell Peppers

Preparation time: 15 minutes

Cooking time: 25 minutes

Servings: 4

Ingredients:

- 4 bell peppers, that is halved and seeds removed
- 2 cups broccoli florets, steamed
- 1 cup shredded cheddar cheese
- 1/2 cup cream cheese, softened
- 1/4 cup grated Parmesan cheese
- 2 cloves garlic, minced
- 1 tsp dried thyme
- Salt and pepper to taste
- Fresh parsley for garnish

Directions:

1. Preheat the oven to 375°F.

2. In your bowl, combine steamed broccoli, shredded cheddar cheese, cream cheese, grated Parmesan, minced garlic, dried thyme, salt, and pepper.

3. Fill each bell pepper half with the broccoli and cheese mixture.

4. Place stuffed peppers in a baking dish then bake for 25 minutes or 'til the peppers are tender.

5. Garnish using fresh parsley before serving.

Per serving: Calories: 280kcal; Fat: 20g; Protein: 10g; Carbs: 15g; Sugar: 6g; Fiber: 5g

Mediterranean Zucchini Boats

Preparation time: 20 minutes

Cooking time: 25 minutes

Servings: 4

Ingredients:

- 4 large zucchinis, halved lengthwise
- 1 cup cherry tomatoes, halved
- 1/2 cup black olives, sliced
- 1/2 cup crumbled feta cheese
- 2 tbsp olive oil
- 2 cloves garlic, minced
- 1 tsp dried oregano
- Salt and pepper to taste
- Fresh parsley for garnish

Directions:

1. Preheat the oven to 375°F.
2. Scoop out the center of each zucchini half, creating a boat shape.
3. In your bowl, mix cherry tomatoes, black olives, crumbled feta, olive oil, minced garlic, dried oregano, salt, and pepper.
4. Fill each zucchini boat with the Mediterranean mixture.
5. Place zucchini boats in a baking dish then bake for 25 minutes or 'til the zucchini is tender.
6. Garnish using fresh parsley before serving.

Per serving: Calories: 180kcal; Fat: 12g; Protein: 6g; Carbs: 15g; Sugar: 8g; Fiber: 5g

Brussel Sprouts and Parmesan Bake

Preparation time: 15 minutes

Cooking time: 25 minutes

Servings: 4

Ingredients:

- 1 lb Brussels sprouts, trimmed and halved
- 2 tbsp olive oil
- 1/4 cup grated Parmesan cheese
- 2 cloves garlic, minced
- 1 tsp dried thyme
- Salt and pepper to taste
- Lemon wedges for serving

Directions:

1. Preheat the oven to 400°F.
2. In your bowl, toss Brussels sprouts with olive oil, grated Parmesan, minced garlic, dried thyme, salt, and pepper.
3. Spread your Brussels sprouts in a single layer on baking sheet.
4. Bake for 25 minutes or 'til golden and crispy.
5. Serve with lemon wedges on the side.

Per serving: Calories: 150kcal; Fat: 10g; Protein: 6g; Carbs: 12g; Sugar: 4g; Fiber: 5g

Low-Carb Dessert Recipes

Keto Chocolate Avocado Mousse

Preparation time: 10 minutes

Cooking time: 0 minutes

Servings: 4

Ingredients:

- 2 ripe avocados, peeled and pitted
- 1/4 cup unsweetened cocoa powder
- 1/4 cup almond milk
- 1/4 cup powdered erythritol (or your preferred low-carb sweetener)
- 1 tsp vanilla extract
- Pinch of salt
- Whipped cream for garnish (optional)

Directions:

1. In your blender or food processor, combine avocados, cocoa powder, almond milk, powdered erythritol, vanilla extract, and a pinch of salt.

2. Blend 'til smooth and creamy.

3. Spoon the mousse into serving glasses then refrigerate for at least 2 hours.

4. Garnish using whipped cream before serving if desired.

Per serving: Calories: 180kcal; Fat: 15g; Protein: 3g; Carbs: 10g; Sugar: 1g; Fiber: 7g

Almond Flour Chocolate Chip Cookies

Preparation time: 15 minutes

Cooking time: 12 minutes

Servings: 12 cookies

Ingredients:

- 2 cups almond flour
- 1/4 cup coconut oil, melted
- 1/4 cup powdered erythritol (or your preferred low-carb sweetener)
- 1 tsp vanilla extract
- 1/4 tsp baking soda
- Pinch of salt
- 1/2 cup sugar-free chocolate chips

Directions:

1. Preheat the oven to 350 deg. F then line your baking sheet using parchment paper.

2. In your bowl, combine almond flour, melted coconut oil, powdered erythritol, vanilla extract, baking soda, and a pinch of salt.

3. Fold in sugar-free chocolate chips.

4. Scoop tablespoon-sized portions of dough onto your prepared baking sheet.

5. Bake for 10-12 minutes or 'til the edges are golden.

6. Let cookies to cool on your baking sheet before transferring to a wire rack.

Per serving: Calories: 150kcal; Fat: 12g; Protein: 3g; Carbs: 6g; Sugar: 1g; Fiber: 2g

Berry and Cream Cheese Fat Bombs

Preparation time: 10 minutes

Cooking time: 0 minutes

Servings: 8 fat bombs

Ingredients:

- 1/2 cup cream cheese, softened
- 1/4 cup coconut oil, melted
- 1/2 cup mixed berries (blueberries, raspberries, strawberries), chopped
- 2 tbsp powdered erythritol (or your preferred low-carb sweetener)
- 1/2 tsp vanilla extract

Directions:

1. In your bowl, beat together softened cream cheese, melted coconut oil, powdered erythritol, and vanilla extract 'til smooth.

2. Gently fold in the chopped mixed berries.

3. Spoon mixture into silicone molds or an ice cube tray.

4. Freeze for at least 2 hours or 'til firm.

5. Pop fat bombs out of the molds then store in the freezer.

Per serving: Calories: 90kcal; Fat: 8g; Protein: 1g; Carbs: 2g; Sugar: 1g; Fiber: 1g

Coconut Flour Lemon Poppy Seed Muffins

Preparation time: 15 minutes

Cooking time: 20 minutes

Servings: 8 muffins

Ingredients:

- 1/2 cup coconut flour
- 1/4 cup almond flour
- 1/4 cup powdered erythritol (or your preferred low-carb sweetener)
- 1/2 tsp baking powder
- 1/4 tsp salt
- 1/4 cup coconut oil, melted
- 4 large eggs
- 1/4 cup unsweetened almond milk
- Zest and juice of 1 lemon
- 1 tbsp poppy seeds

Directions:

1. Preheat the oven to 350 deg. F then line a muffin tin using paper liners.

2. In your bowl, whisk together coconut flour, almond flour, powdered erythritol, baking powder, and salt.

3. In your separate bowl, beat together melted coconut oil, eggs, almond milk, lemon zest, and lemon juice.

4. Combine your wet and dry ingredients, then fold in poppy seeds.

5. Divide batter evenly among your muffin cups.

6. Bake for 20 minutes or 'til a toothpick inserted into the center comes out clean.

7. Let the muffins to cool in the tin before transferring to a wire rack.

Per serving: Calories: 120kcal; Fat: 9g; Protein: 4g; Carbs: 5g; Sugar: 1g; Fiber: 3g

Dark Chocolate and Almond Bark

Preparation time: 10 minutes

Cooking time: 0 minutes

Servings: 8

Ingredients:

- 1 cup dark chocolate chips (70% cocoa)
- 1/2 cup almonds, chopped
- 1/4 tsp sea salt

Directions:

1. Line a baking sheet using parchment paper.

2. In your microwave-safe bowl, melt the dark chocolate chips in 30second intervals, stirring among each interval 'til smooth.

3. Pour melted chocolate onto your prepared baking sheet, spreading it into an even layer.

4. Sprinkle chopped almonds evenly over the melted chocolate.

5. Sprinkle sea salt over the top.

6. Refrigerate for at least 1 hour or 'til the chocolate is set.

7. Once set, break into pieces.

Per serving: Calories: 150kcal; Fat: 10g; Protein: 3g; Carbs: 15g; Sugar: 8g; Fiber: 3g

Avocado Chocolate Pudding

Preparation time: 10 minutes

Cooking time: 0 minutes

Servings: 4

Ingredients:

- 2 ripe avocados, peeled and pitted
- 1/4 cup unsweetened cocoa powder
- 1/4 cup almond milk
- 1/4 cup powdered erythritol (or your preferred low-carb sweetener)
- 1 tsp vanilla extract
- Pinch of salt
- Whipped cream for garnish (optional)

Directions:

1. In your blender or food processor, combine avocados, cocoa powder, almond milk, powdered erythritol, vanilla extract, and a pinch of salt.

2. Blend 'til smooth and creamy.

3. Spoon the pudding into serving glasses then refrigerate for at least 2 hours.

4. Garnish using whipped cream before serving if desired.

Per serving: Calories: 180kcal; Fat: 15g; Protein: 3g; Carbs: 10g; Sugar: 1g; Fiber: 7g

Keto Cheesecake Bites

Preparation time: 15 minutes

Cooking time: 0 minutes

Servings: 12 bites

Ingredients:

- 8 oz cream cheese, softened
- 1/4 cup powdered erythritol (or your preferred low-carb sweetener)
- 1 tsp vanilla extract
- 1/2 cup almond flour
- 1/4 cup melted butter
- Sugar-free fruit preserves for topping (optional)

Directions:

1. In your bowl, beat together softened cream cheese, powdered erythritol, and vanilla extract 'til smooth.

2. In your separate bowl, combine almond flour and melted butter.

3. Add almond flour mixture to the cream cheese mixture and mix until well combined.

4. Scoop tablespoon-sized portions of the mixture then roll into balls.

5. Place the cheesecake bites on a parchment-lined tray then refrigerate for at least 2 hours.

6. Optionally, top each bite with sugar-free fruit preserves before serving.

Per serving: Calories: 120kcal; Fat: 10g; Protein: 3g; Carbs: 5g; Sugar: 1g; Fiber: 1g

Almond Flour Blueberry Muffins

Preparation time: 15 minutes

Cooking time: 20 minutes

Servings: 8 muffins

Ingredients:

- 1 cup almond flour
- 1/4 cup coconut flour
- 1/4 cup powdered erythritol (or your preferred low-carb sweetener)
- 1/2 tsp baking powder
- 1/4 tsp salt
- 1/4 cup melted coconut oil
- 3 large eggs
- 1/4 cup unsweetened almond milk
- 1 tsp vanilla extract
- 1/2 cup fresh blueberries

Directions:

1. Preheat the oven to 350 deg. F then line a muffin tin using paper liners.

2. In your bowl, whisk together almond flour, coconut flour, powdered erythritol, baking powder, and salt.

3. In your separate bowl, whisk together melted coconut oil, eggs, almond milk, and vanilla extract.

4. Combine your wet and dry ingredients, then fold in fresh blueberries.

5. Divide batter evenly among your muffin cups.

6. Bake for 20 minutes or 'til a toothpick inserted into the center comes out clean.

7. Let the muffins to cool in the tin before transferring to a wire rack.

Per serving: Calories: 180kcal; Fat: 15g; Protein: 6g; Carbs: 6g; Sugar: 2g; Fiber: 2g

Chocolate Peanut Butter Fat Bombs

Preparation time: 10 minutes

Cooking time: 0 minutes

Servings: 12 fat bombs

Ingredients:

- 1/2 cup coconut oil, melted
- 1/4 cup unsweetened cocoa powder
- 1/4 cup powdered erythritol (or your preferred low-carb sweetener)
- 1/2 cup creamy peanut butter
- 1 tsp vanilla extract
- Pinch of salt

Directions:

1. In your bowl, whisk together melted coconut oil, cocoa powder, powdered erythritol, peanut butter, vanilla extract, and a pinch of salt.

2. Spoon mixture into silicone molds or an ice cube tray.

3. Freeze for at least 2 hours or 'til firm.

4. Pop fat bombs out of the molds then store in the freezer.

Per serving: Calories: 130kcal; Fat: 12g; Protein: 3g; Carbs: 3g; Sugar: 1g; Fiber: 1g

Vanilla Coconut Flour Mug Cake

Preparation time: 5 minutes

Cooking time: 2 minutes

Servings: 1 mug cake

Ingredients:

- 2 tbsp coconut flour
- 1 tbsp powdered erythritol (or your preferred low-carb sweetener)
- 1/4 tsp baking powder
- Pinch of salt
- 2 tbsp melted coconut oil
- 2 tbsp unsweetened almond milk
- 1/2 tsp vanilla extract

Directions:

1. In your microwave-safe mug, whisk together coconut flour, powdered erythritol, baking powder, and a pinch of salt.

2. Add melted coconut oil, almond milk, and vanilla extract. Mix 'til smooth.

3. Microwave on high for 2 minutes or 'til the cake is firm then cooked through.

4. Let the mug cake to cool for a minute before serving.

Per serving: Calories: 260kcal; Fat: 22g; Protein: 4g; Carbs: 10g; Sugar: 2g; Fiber: 6g

Raspberry Coconut Chia Seed Pudding

Preparation time: 10 minutes

Cooking time: 0 minutes

Servings: 2

Ingredients:

- 1/4 cup chia seeds
- 1 cup unsweetened coconut milk
- 1/2 tsp vanilla extract
- 1 tbsp powdered erythritol (or your preferred low-carb sweetener)
- 1/2 cup fresh raspberries
- Unsweetened shredded coconut for garnish

Directions:

1. In your bowl, whisk together chia seeds, coconut milk, vanilla extract, and powdered erythritol.
2. Let the mixture sit for 5 minutes, then whisk again to prevent clumping.
3. Cover then refrigerate for at least 4 hours or overnight.
4. Before serving, stir the pudding to ensure a consistent texture.
5. Spoon the chia seed pudding into serving glasses, layering with fresh raspberries.
6. Garnish using unsweetened shredded coconut.

Per serving: Calories: 180kcal; Fat: 14g; Protein: 3g; Carbs: 14g; Sugar: 2g; Fiber: 9g

Low-Carb Snack and Drink Recipes

Parmesan Crisps

Preparation time: 5 minutes

Cooking time: 7 minutes

Servings: 12

Ingredients:

- 1 cup grated Parmesan cheese

Directions:

1. Preheat the oven to 400 deg. F then line your baking sheet using parchment paper.
2. Drop tablespoon-sized portions of grated Parmesan onto your baking sheet, leaving space between each.
3. Flatten each portion slightly to form a thin, even layer.
4. Bake for 5-7 minutes or 'til the edges are golden and crisp.
5. Let the Parmesan crisps to cool before removing them from the baking sheet.

Per serving: Calories: 100kcal; Fat: 7g; Protein: 10g; Carbs: 1g; Sugar: 0g; Fiber: 0g

Almond and Coconut Energy Bites

Preparation time: 15 minutes

Cooking time: 0 minutes

Servings: 12

Ingredients:

- 1 cup almond flour
- 1/2 cup unsweetened shredded coconut
- 1/4 cup almond butter
- 2 tbsp coconut oil, melted
- 1 tbsp chia seeds
- 1 tbsp powdered erythritol (or your preferred low-carb sweetener)
- 1/2 tsp vanilla extract
- Pinch of salt

Directions:

1. In your bowl, combine vanilla extract, almond flour, shredded coconut, almond butter, melted coconut oil, chia seeds, powdered erythritol, and a pinch of salt.

2. Mix until well combined.

3. Roll mixture into tablespoon-sized balls and place them on a parchment-lined tray.

4. Refrigerate for at least 30 minutes before serving.

Per serving: Calories: 120kcal; Fat: 10g; Protein: 3g; Carbs: 4g; Sugar: 1g; Fiber: 2g

Spicy Roasted Chickpeas

Preparation time: 10 minutes

Cooking time: 40 minutes

Servings: 4

Ingredients:

- 2 cans (15 oz each) chickpeas, that is drained and rinsed
- 2 tbsp olive oil
- 1 tsp smoked paprika
- 1/2 tsp cayenne pepper
- 1/2 tsp garlic powder
- 1/2 tsp cumin
- Salt to taste

Directions:

1. Preheat the oven to 400 deg. F then line your baking sheet using parchment paper.

2. Pat your chickpeas dry using a paper towel and place them on your baking sheet.

3. Drizzle olive oil over the chickpeas then toss to coat.

4. In your small bowl, mix smoked paprika, cayenne pepper, garlic powder, cumin, and salt.

5. Sprinkle the spice mixture over the chickpeas then toss to coat evenly.

6. Roast in to your oven for 40 minutes, shaking the pan occasionally for even cooking.

7. Let the roasted chickpeas cool before serving.

Per serving: Calories: 180kcal; Fat: 7g; Protein: 7g; Carbs: 23g; Sugar: 4g; Fiber: 6g

Keto Deviled Eggs

Preparation time: 15 minutes

Cooking time: 0 minutes

Servings: 12

Ingredients:

- 6 hard-boiled eggs, that is peeled and cut in half
- 3 tbsp mayonnaise
- 1 tsp Dijon mustard
- 1/2 tsp white wine vinegar
- Salt and pepper to taste
- Paprika for garnish

Directions:

1. Scoop egg yolks into your bowl and mash them using a fork.
2. Add mayonnaise, Dijon mustard, white wine vinegar, salt, and pepper. Mix 'til smooth.
3. Spoon or pipe the filling back into your egg whites.
4. Sprinkle using paprika for garnish.
5. Refrigerate until ready to serve.

Per serving: Calories: 100kcal; Fat: 8g; Protein: 6g; Carbs: 1g; Sugar: 0g; Fiber: 0g

Bacon-Wrapped Asparagus Spears

Preparation time: 10 minutes

Cooking time: 15 minutes

Servings: 4

Ingredients:

- 1 bunch asparagus, tough ends trimmed
- 8 slices bacon, cut in half
- Olive oil for brushing
- Salt and pepper to taste

Directions:

1. Preheat the oven to 400 deg. F then line your baking sheet using parchment paper.
2. Wrap each asparagus spear with half a slice of bacon, spiraling it along the length.
3. Place the bacon-wrapped asparagus on your baking sheet.
4. Brush with olive oil then season using salt and pepper.
5. Bake for 15 minutes or 'til the bacon is crispy.
6. Serve warm.

Per serving: Calories: 150kcal; Fat: 11g; Protein: 8g; Carbs: 5g; Sugar: 2g; Fiber: 2g

Avocado and Bacon Dip

Preparation time: 15 minutes

Cooking time: 0 minutes

Servings: 6

Ingredients:

- 2 ripe avocados, peeled and pitted
- 6 slices bacon, cooked and crumbled
- 1/4 cup sour cream
- 1/4 cup mayonnaise
- 1/4 cup diced red onion
- 1 clove garlic, minced
- 1 tbsp fresh lime juice
- Salt and pepper to taste
- Chopped fresh cilantro for garnish (optional)

Directions:

1. In your bowl, mash the avocados using a fork.
2. Add crumbled bacon, sour cream, mayonnaise, red onion, minced garlic, lime juice, salt, and pepper. Mix until well combined.
3. Garnish using chopped fresh cilantro if desired.
4. Serve with low-carb vegetable sticks or crispy Parmesan crisps.

Per serving: Calories: 180kcal; Fat: 16g; Protein: 4g; Carbs: 6g; Sugar: 1g; Fiber: 4g

Iced Herbal Mint Tea

Preparation time: 5 minutes

Cooking time: 0 minutes

Servings: 4

Ingredients:

- 4 cups water
- 4 herbal mint tea bags
- 1 tbsp fresh mint leaves, chopped
- 1 tbsp powdered erythritol (or your preferred low-carb sweetener)
- Ice cubes
- Lemon slices for garnish (optional)

Directions:

1. Boil 4 cups of water.
2. Add the herbal mint tea bags to the boiling water and steep for 5 minutes.
3. Remove the tea bags and stir in fresh mint leaves and powdered erythritol.
4. Let the tea cool to room temperature, then refrigerate for at least 2 hours.
5. Serve over ice then garnish with lemon slices if desired.

Per serving: Calories: 0kcal; Fat: 0g; Protein: 0g; Carbs: 0g; Sugar: 0g; Fiber: 0g

Preparation time: 10 minutes

Cooking time: 0 minutes

Servings: 4

Ingredients:

- 2 cups unsweetened almond milk
- 1/2 cup chia seeds
- 1 tbsp powdered erythritol (or your preferred low-carb sweetener)
- 1/2 tsp vanilla extract
- Fresh berries for topping

Directions:

1. In your bowl, whisk together almond milk, chia seeds, powdered erythritol, and vanilla extract.

2. Cover then refrigerate for at least 4 hours or overnight, stirring occasionally to prevent clumping.

3. Serve chia seed pudding in individual bowls and top with fresh berries.

Per serving: Calories: 70kcal; Fat: 5g; Protein: 2g; Carbs: 6g; Sugar: 0g; Fiber: 4g

Chapter 8: High-Carb Recipes

High-Carb Breakfast Recipes

Classic Oatmeal with Fresh Fruits

Preparation time: 5 minutes

Cooking time: 5 minutes

Servings: 1

Ingredients:

- 1/2 cup old-fashioned oats
- 1 cup milk (dairy or plant-based)
- 1/2 banana, sliced
- Handful of berries (strawberries, blueberries, or raspberries)
- 1 tablespoon honey
- 1 tablespoon chopped nuts (almonds, walnuts, or pecans)

Directions:

1. In your saucepan, bring the milk to a simmer.

2. Stir in the oats then cook for 5 minutes, or 'til the desired consistency is reached.

3. Transfer the oatmeal to a bowl and top with banana slices, berries, honey, and chopped nuts.

Per serving: Calories: 350kcal; Fat: 10g; Protein: 12g; Carbs: 55g; Sugar: 20g; Fiber: 7g

Whole Grain Pancakes with Maple Syrup

Preparation time: 10 minutes

Cooking time: 10 minutes

Servings: 2

Ingredients:

- 1 cup whole grain pancake mix
- 3/4 cup water
- 1/2 banana, mashed
- 2 tablespoons maple syrup
- Fresh berries for topping

Directions:

1. In your bowl, mix the pancake mix, water, and mashed banana until well combined.

2. Heat a non-stick skillet in medium heat then place 1/4 cup of batter for each pancake.

3. Cook 'til bubbles form on the surface, then flip then cook 'til golden brown.

4. Serve with maple syrup and fresh berries.

Per serving: Calories: 320kcal; Fat: 2g; Protein: 6g; Carbs: 70g; Sugar: 18g; Fiber: 8g

Berry and Yogurt Parfait

Preparation time: 10 minutes

Cooking time: 0 minutes

Servings: 1

Ingredients:

- 1 cup Greek yogurt
- 1/2 cup granola
- 1/2 cup mixed berries (strawberries, blueberries, and raspberries)
- 1 tablespoon honey

Directions:

1. In your glass or bowl, layer Greek yogurt, granola, and mixed berries.
2. Drizzle honey on top.
3. Repeat the layers then finish with a dollop of yogurt and a few berries on top.

Per serving: Calories: 380kcal; Fat: 10g; Protein: 20g; Carbs: 55g; Sugar: 22g; Fiber: 7g

Sweet Potato Hash with Eggs

Preparation time: 15 minutes

Cooking time: 20 minutes

Servings: 2

Ingredients:

- 2 medium sweet potatoes, peeled and diced
- 1 bell pepper, chopped
- 1 onion, diced
- 2 tablespoons olive oil
- Salt and pepper to taste
- 4 eggs
- Fresh parsley for garnish

Directions:

1. In your skillet, heat olive oil in medium heat. Add sweet potatoes, bell pepper, and onion. Season using salt and pepper.
2. Cook 'til sweet potatoes are tender and lightly browned, about 15-20 minutes.
3. Create four wells in your hash then crack an egg into each. Cover then cook 'til the eggs are set.
4. Garnish using fresh parsley then serve.

Per serving: Calories: 380kcal; Fat: 18g; Protein: 14g; Carbs: 45g; Sugar: 10g; Fiber: 7g

Blueberry Almond Butter Smoothie Bowl

Preparation time: 10 minutes

Cooking time: 0 minutes

Servings: 1

Ingredients:

- 1 cup frozen blueberries
- 1 banana
- 1/2 cup almond milk
- 2 tablespoons almond butter
- Granola for topping
- Chia seeds for garnish

Directions:

1. In your blender, combine frozen blueberries, banana, almond milk, and almond butter. Blend 'til smooth.

2. Pour the smoothie into your bowl and top with granola and chia seeds.

Per serving: Calories: 420kcal; Fat: 22g; Protein: 10g; Carbs: 55g; Sugar: 25g; Fiber: 10g

Apple Cinnamon Quinoa Porridge

Preparation time: 15 minutes

Cooking time: 15 minutes

Servings: 2

Ingredients:

- 1 cup quinoa, rinsed
- 2 cups unsweetened almond milk
- 1 apple, diced
- 1 teaspoon cinnamon
- 1 tablespoon maple syrup
- Chopped nuts for topping

Directions:

1. In your saucepan, combine quinoa, almond milk, diced apple, and cinnamon. Bring to a simmer.

2. Simmer for 15 minutes or 'til quinoa is cooked and the mixture thickens.

3. Stir in maple syrup then serve topped with chopped nuts.

Per serving: Calories: 320kcal; Fat: 8g; Protein: 10g; Carbs: 55g; Sugar: 15g; Fiber: 6g

Tropical Fruit Salad with Honey Drizzle

Preparation time: 15 minutes

Cooking time: 0 minutes

Servings: 4

Ingredients:

- 2 cups pineapple, diced
- 1 cup mango, diced
- 1 cup kiwi, sliced
- 1 cup strawberries, halved
- 2 tablespoons honey
- Fresh mint for garnish

Directions:

1. In your large bowl, combine pineapple, mango, kiwi, and strawberries.

2. Drizzle honey over the fruit then toss gently to coat.

3. Garnish using fresh mint before serving.

Per serving: Calories: 120kcal; Fat: 1g; Protein: 2g; Carbs: 30g; Sugar: 20g; Fiber: 4g

Brown Sugar and Cinnamon French Toast

Preparation time: 10 minutes

Cooking time: 10 minutes

Servings: 2

Ingredients:

- 4 slices whole grain bread or rye bread
- 2 large eggs
- 1/2 cup milk (dairy or plant-based)
- 1 teaspoon vanilla extract
- 2 tablespoons brown sugar
- 1 teaspoon ground cinnamon
- Butter for cooking

Directions:

1. In your shallow bowl, whisk together eggs, milk, vanilla extract, brown sugar, and cinnamon.

2. Heat your skillet in medium heat and add a small amount of butter.

3. Dip each slice of your bread into egg mixture, ensuring it's coated evenly, then cook 'til golden brown on both sides.

4. Serve with a sprinkle of your extra cinnamon and a drizzle of maple syrup.

Per serving: Calories: 350kcal; Fat: 10g; Protein: 12g; Carbs: 55g; Sugar: 15g; Fiber: 6g

Peanut Butter Banana Breakfast Wrap

Preparation time: 5 minutes

Cooking time: 5 minutes

Servings: 1

Ingredients:

- 1 whole grain tortilla
- 2 tablespoons peanut butter
- 1 banana, sliced
- 1 tablespoon honey
- 1 tablespoon chopped nuts (optional)

Directions:

1. Spread peanut butter evenly over the tortilla.
2. Place banana slices on one half of the tortilla and drizzle with honey.
3. Fold the tortilla in half, creating a wrap.
4. Optional: Warm the wrap in your skillet for a minute on each side.
5. Sprinkle using chopped nuts if desired before serving.

Per serving: Calories: 450kcal; Fat: 20g; Protein: 10g; Carbs: 60g; Sugar: 25g; Fiber: 8g

High-Carb Beef, Pork, and Poultry Recipes

Beef and Vegetable Stir-Fry with Brown Rice

Preparation time: 15 minutes

Cooking time: 15 minutes

Servings: 4

Ingredients:

- 1 lb lean beef, that is thinly sliced
- 2 cups broccoli florets
- 1 bell pepper, sliced
- 1 carrot, julienned
- 2 tablespoons soy sauce
- 1 tablespoon oyster sauce
- 1 tablespoon sesame oil
- 2 cups cooked brown rice

Directions:

1. In your wok or skillet, heat sesame oil in medium-high heat.
2. Add beef slices and stir-fry until browned. Remove from the wok.
3. Stir-fry broccoli, bell pepper, and carrot until tender-crisp.
4. Add cooked beef back to the wok, pour in soy sauce and oyster sauce. Stir until everything is well coated.
5. Serve over cooked brown rice.

Per serving: Calories: 400kcal; Fat: 12g; Protein: 25g; Carbs: 50g; Sugar: 4g; Fiber: 7g

Orange Glazed Chicken with Sweet Potatoes

Preparation time: 20 minutes

Cooking time: 30 minutes

Servings: 4

Ingredients:

- 4 boneless, skinless chicken breasts
- 2 sweet potatoes, peeled and diced
- 1/2 cup orange juice
- 2 tablespoons honey
- 1 tablespoon olive oil
- 1 teaspoon ground ginger
- Salt and pepper to taste

Directions:

1. Preheat the oven to 400°F.
2. Season chicken breasts with salt, pepper, and ground ginger.
3. In your bowl, mix orange juice and honey.
4. Place chicken breasts and sweet potatoes on your baking sheet. Drizzle using olive oil then pour the orange-honey mixture over.
5. Bake for 25-30 minutes or 'til chicken is cooked through and sweet potatoes are tender.

Per serving: Calories: 380kcal; Fat: 8g; Protein: 30g; Carbs: 50g; Sugar: 20g; Fiber: 6g

BBQ Pulled Pork Sandwiches

Preparation time: 10 minutes

Cooking time: 4 hours (slow cooker)

Servings: 6

Ingredients:

- 2 lbs pork shoulder
- 1 cup BBQ sauce
- 1 onion, sliced
- 6 whole grain hamburger buns
- Coleslaw for topping

Directions:

1. Place pork shoulder and sliced onions in a slow cooker. Pour BBQ sauce over the pork.
2. Cook on low for 4-6 hours 'til pork is tender and easily shredded.
3. Shred pork using two forks and mix with the sauce.
4. Serve on whole grain buns, topped with coleslaw.

Per serving: Calories: 450kcal; Fat: 15g; Protein: 25g; Carbs: 55g; Sugar: 20g; Fiber: 8g

Teriyaki Chicken Skewers with Jasmine Rice

Preparation time: 15 minutes

Cooking time: 15 minutes

Servings: 4

Ingredients:

- 1.5 lbs boneless, that is skinless chicken thighs, cut into cubes
- 1/2 cup teriyaki sauce
- 1 tablespoon honey
- 2 bell peppers, cut into chunks
- 1 red onion, cut into chunks
- 2 cups cooked jasmine rice

Directions:

1. In your bowl, combine chicken cubes with teriyaki sauce and honey. Let it marinate for 10 minutes.

2. Thread marinated chicken, bell peppers, and red onion onto skewers.

3. Grill or broil the skewers for 10-12 minutes, turning occasionally, until chicken is fully cooked.

4. Serve over cooked jasmine rice.

Per serving: Calories: 420kcal; Fat: 10g; Protein: 30g; Carbs: 55g; Sugar: 10g; Fiber: 3g

Beef and Broccoli with Noodles

Preparation time: 15 minutes

Cooking time: 20 minutes

Servings: 4

Ingredients:

- 8 oz whole wheat noodles
- 1 lb flank steak, that is thinly sliced
- 2 cups broccoli florets
- 3 tablespoons soy sauce
- 1 tablespoon oyster sauce
- 2 tablespoons hoisin sauce
- 2 cloves garlic, minced
- 1 tablespoon sesame oil

Directions:

1. Cook noodles according to package instructions.

2. In your wok or skillet, heat sesame oil in medium-high heat. Add sliced flank steak then cook 'til browned.

3. Add broccoli and minced garlic, stir-frying until broccoli is tender-crisp.

4. In your small bowl, mix soy sauce, oyster sauce, and hoisin sauce. Pour over the beef and broccoli, stirring until well combined.

5. Serve the beef and broccoli over cooked noodles.

Per serving: Calories: 450kcal; Fat: 12g; Protein: 30g; Carbs: 55g; Sugar: 4g; Fiber: 8g

Chicken Fajita Burrito Bowl

Preparation time: 15 minutes

Cooking time: 20 minutes

Servings: 4

Ingredients:

- 1 lb boneless, skinless chicken breasts, sliced
- 1 bell pepper, sliced
- 1 onion, sliced
- 2 tablespoons fajita seasoning
- 1 cup cooked brown rice
- 1 cup black beans, that is drained and rinsed
- 1 cup corn kernels
- Salsa and guacamole for topping

Directions:

1. In your skillet, cook sliced chicken with fajita seasoning until browned.

2. Add sliced bell pepper and onion to your skillet, cooking 'til vegetables are tender.

3. In serving bowls, layer cooked brown rice, black beans, corn, and the chicken and vegetable mixture.

4. Top with salsa and guacamole before serving.

Per serving: Calories: 420kcal; Fat: 8g; Protein: 30g; Carbs: 60g; Sugar: 5g; Fiber: 10g

Sweet and Sour Meatballs with Quinoa

Preparation time: 20 minutes

Cooking time: 20 minutes

Servings: 4

Ingredients:

- 1 lb ground beef
- 1/2 cup breadcrumbs
- 1 egg
- 1 cup pineapple chunks (fresh or canned)
- 1 bell pepper, diced
- 1/2 cup sweet and sour sauce
- 1 cup cooked quinoa

Directions:

1. In your bowl, mix ground beef, breadcrumbs, and egg. Form into meatballs.

2. In your skillet, cook meatballs until browned then cooked through.

3. In the same skillet, add pineapple chunks, diced bell pepper, and sweet and sour sauce. Cook 'til heated through.

4. Serve meatballs and sauce over cooked quinoa.

Per serving: Calories: 450kcal; Fat: 20g; Protein: 25g; Carbs: 45g; Sugar: 15g; Fiber: 5g

Chili Lime Grilled Chicken Tacos

Preparation time: 15 minutes

Cooking time: 15 minutes

Servings: 4

Ingredients:

- 1.5 lbs boneless, skinless chicken breasts
- Zest and juice of 2 limes
- 2 tablespoons olive oil
- 2 teaspoons chili powder
- 1 teaspoon cumin
- 1 teaspoon garlic powder
- Salt and pepper to taste
- 8 small corn tortillas
- Sliced cabbage and cilantro for topping

Directions:

1. In your bowl, mix lime zest, lime juice, olive oil, chili powder, cumin, garlic powder, salt, and pepper.

2. Marinate chicken in the mixture for at least 15 minutes.

3. Grill chicken until fully cooked, then slice into strips.

4. Warm corn tortillas and fill with grilled chicken strips. Top with sliced cabbage and cilantro.

Per serving: Calories: 380kcal; Fat: 12g; Protein: 30g; Carbs: 35g; Sugar: 2g; Fiber: 5g

Pork and Pineapple Skewers with Coconut Rice

Preparation time: 20 minutes

Cooking time: 20 minutes

Servings: 4

Ingredients:

- 1 lb pork tenderloin, cut into cubes
- 1 cup pineapple chunks
- 1 cup jasmine rice
- 1 can (14 oz) coconut milk
- 2 tablespoons soy sauce
- 1 tablespoon honey
- Wooden skewers, soaked in water

Directions:

1. Thread pork cubes and pineapple chunks onto skewers.

2. In your bowl, mix soy sauce and honey. Brush over skewers.

3. Grill skewers until pork is cooked through.

4. In your saucepan, combine jasmine rice and coconut milk. Cook according to package instructions.

5. Serve skewers over coconut rice.

Per serving: Calories: 480kcal; Fat: 20g; Protein: 25g; Carbs: 55g; Sugar: 10g; Fiber: 2g

Italian Style Beef and Pasta

Preparation time: 15 minutes

Cooking time: 20 minutes

Servings: 4

Ingredients:

- 1 lb lean ground beef
- 8 oz whole wheat pasta
- 1 can (14 oz) diced tomatoes, undrained
- 1 teaspoon dried oregano
- 1 teaspoon dried basil
- 2 cloves garlic, minced
- Salt and pepper to taste
- Grated Parmesan cheese for topping

Directions:

1. Cook pasta according to package instructions.

2. In your skillet, brown ground beef. Drain excess fat.

3. Add diced tomatoes (with juice), oregano, basil, garlic, salt, and pepper to your skillet. Simmer for 10 minutes.

4. Toss cooked pasta with the beef and tomato mixture.

5. Serve topped with grated Parmesan cheese.

Per serving: Calories: 420kcal; Fat: 10g; Protein: 30g; Carbs: 55g; Sugar: 5g; Fiber: 8g

Lemon Herb Chicken with Roasted Potatoes

Preparation time: 15 minutes

Cooking time: 40 minutes

Servings: 4

Ingredients:

- 4 bone-in, skin-on chicken thighs
- 1 lb baby potatoes, halved
- Zest and juice of 1 lemon
- 2 tablespoons olive oil
- 2 teaspoons dried rosemary
- 1 teaspoon dried thyme
- Salt and pepper to taste

Directions:

1. Preheat the oven to 400°F.

2. In your bowl, mix lemon zest, lemon juice, olive oil, rosemary, thyme, salt, and pepper.

3. Toss chicken thighs and halved potatoes in the lemon herb mixture.

4. Roast in to your oven for 40 minutes or 'til the chicken is cooked through and potatoes are golden.

Per serving: Calories: 450kcal; Fat: 20g; Protein: 30g; Carbs: 35g; Sugar: 2g; Fiber: 5g

Balsamic Glazed Beef with Pasta

Preparation time: 15 minutes

Cooking time: 20 minutes

Servings: 4

Ingredients:

- 1 lb sirloin steak, that is thinly sliced
- 8 oz whole wheat pasta
- 1/4 cup balsamic vinegar
- 2 tablespoons soy sauce
- 1 tablespoon honey
- 2 cloves garlic, minced
- 1 tablespoon olive oil
- Cherry tomatoes and fresh basil for garnish

Directions:

1. Cook pasta according to package instructions.

2. In your skillet, heat olive oil in medium-high heat. Add sliced sirloin then cook 'til browned.

3. In your bowl, whisk together balsamic vinegar, soy sauce, honey, and minced garlic. Pour over the beef then simmer 'til the sauce thickens.

4. Toss cooked pasta with the balsamic glazed beef.

5. Garnish using cherry tomatoes and fresh basil.

Per serving: Calories: 420kcal; Fat: 12g; Protein: 30g; Carbs: 55g; Sugar: 8g; Fiber: 8g

High-Carb Fish and Seafood Recipes

Lemon Garlic Butter Shrimp with Linguine

Preparation time: 15 minutes

Cooking time: 15 minutes

Servings: 4

Ingredients:

- 8 oz linguine pasta
- 1 lb large shrimp, peeled and deveined
- 3 tablespoons unsalted butter
- 4 cloves garlic, minced
- Zest and juice of 1 lemon
- Salt and pepper to taste
- Fresh parsley for garnish

Directions:

1. Cook linguine according to package instructions.

2. In your large skillet, melt butter in medium heat. Add minced garlic then sauté until fragrant.

3. Add shrimp to your skillet then cook 'til pink and opaque.

4. Stir in lemon zest and juice. Season using salt and pepper.

5. Toss the cooked linguine with the lemon garlic butter shrimp. Garnish using fresh parsley before serving.

Per serving: Calories: 420kcal; Fat: 15g; Protein: 25g; Carbs: 55g; Sugar: 2g; Fiber: 3g

Baked Salmon with Sweet Potato Mash

Preparation time: 20 minutes

Cooking time: 20 minutes

Servings: 4

Ingredients:

- 4 salmon fillets
- 2 large sweet potatoes, peeled and diced
- 2 tablespoons olive oil
- 1 teaspoon garlic powder
- Salt and pepper to taste
- Fresh dill for garnish

Directions:

1. Preheat the oven to 400°F.

2. Place sweet potato cubes on your baking sheet, drizzle with olive oil, then season using garlic powder, salt, and pepper.

3. Bake for 20 minutes or 'til sweet potatoes are tender.

4. Season salmon fillets using salt and pepper, then bake for 15-20 minutes until cooked through.

5. Mash the baked sweet potatoes then serve alongside the baked salmon. Garnish using fresh dill.

Per serving: Calories: 450kcal; Fat: 20g; Protein: 30g; Carbs: 35g; Sugar: 8g; Fiber: 5g

Tuna and Brown Rice Casserole

Preparation time: 15 minutes

Cooking time: 30 minutes

Servings: 6

Ingredients:

- 2 cups cooked brown rice
- 2 cans (5 oz each) tuna, drained
- 1 cup frozen peas
- 1 cup diced carrots
- 1/2 cup plain Greek yogurt
- 1/4 cup mayonnaise
- 1 teaspoon Dijon mustard
- Salt and pepper to taste
- 1 cup shredded cheddar cheese

Directions:

1. Preheat the oven to 375°F.

2. In your large bowl, combine cooked brown rice, tuna, frozen peas, and diced carrots.

3. In your separate bowl, mix Greek yogurt, mayonnaise, Dijon mustard, salt, and pepper.

4. Combine the yogurt mixture with the rice and tuna mixture. Transfer to a baking dish.

5. Top using shredded cheddar cheese then bake for 25-30 minutes or 'til the cheese is melted and bubbly.

Per serving: Calories: 380kcal; Fat: 18g; Protein: 25g; Carbs: 35g; Sugar: 3g; Fiber: 5g

Coconut Curry Shrimp with Basmati Rice

Preparation time: 20 minutes

Cooking time: 20 minutes

Servings: 4

Ingredients:

- 1 lb large shrimp, peeled and deveined
- 1 cup basmati rice
- 1 can (14 oz) coconut milk
- 2 tablespoons red curry paste
- 1 tablespoon olive oil
- 1 onion, finely chopped
- 1 red bell pepper, sliced
- 1 zucchini, sliced
- Salt and pepper to taste
- Fresh cilantro for garnish

Directions:

1. Cook basmati rice according to package instructions.
2. In your large skillet, heat olive oil in medium heat. Add chopped onion then sauté until translucent.
3. Stir in red curry paste then cook for 1-2 minutes.
4. Add coconut milk, sliced red bell pepper, and zucchini. Simmer 'til vegetables are tender.
5. Add shrimp to your skillet then cook 'til pink and opaque. Season using salt and pepper.
6. Serve the coconut curry shrimp over cooked basmati rice. Garnish using fresh cilantro.

Per serving: Calories: 450kcal; Fat: 20g; Protein: 25g; Carbs: 55g; Sugar: 3g; Fiber: 4g

Grilled Tilapia Tacos with Mango Salsa

Preparation time: 20 minutes

Cooking time: 10 minutes

Servings: 4

Ingredients:

- 4 tilapia fillets
- 8 small corn tortillas
- 1 teaspoon cumin
- 1 teaspoon chili powder
- Salt and pepper to taste
- 1 cup diced mango
- 1/2 red onion, finely chopped
- 1 jalapeño, seeded and minced
- Fresh cilantro for garnish
- Lime wedges for serving

Directions:

1. Preheat the grill.
2. Season tilapia fillets with cumin, chili powder, salt, and pepper.
3. Grill tilapia for 4-5 minutes per side until fully cooked.
4. In your bowl, combine diced mango, chopped red onion, minced jalapeño, and fresh cilantro to make the salsa.
5. Assemble tacos with grilled tilapia and mango salsa. Serve with lime wedges.

Per serving: Calories: 320kcal; Fat: 5g; Protein: 25g; Carbs: 45g; Sugar: 10g; Fiber: 6g

Shrimp and Broccoli Stir-Fry with Quinoa

Preparation time: 15 minutes

Cooking time: 15 minutes

Servings: 4

Ingredients:

- 1 lb shrimp, peeled and deveined
- 2 cups broccoli florets
- 1 red bell pepper, sliced
- 1/4 cup soy sauce
- 2 tablespoons hoisin sauce
- 1 tablespoon sesame oil
- 1 tablespoon cornstarch
- 2 tablespoons olive oil
- 2 cups cooked quinoa

Directions:

1. In your bowl, mix soy sauce, hoisin sauce, sesame oil, and cornstarch to create the sauce.

2. Heat olive oil in your wok or skillet over high heat. Add shrimp and stir-fry until pink.

3. Place broccoli and red bell pepper to the wok, stir-frying 'til vegetables are tender-crisp.

4. Place the sauce over the shrimp and vegetables, stirring until everything is coated.

5. Serve over cooked quinoa.

Per serving: Calories: 380kcal; Fat: 15g; Protein: 25g; Carbs: 45g; Sugar: 5g; Fiber: 7g

Creamy Garlic Parmesan Pasta with Scallops

Preparation time: 20 minutes

Cooking time: 15 minutes

Servings: 4

Ingredients:

- 8 oz fettuccine pasta
- 1 lb scallops
- 2 tablespoons butter
- 4 cloves garlic, minced
- 1 cup heavy cream
- 1/2 cup grated Parmesan cheese
- Salt and pepper to taste
- Chopped fresh parsley for garnish

Directions:

1. Cook fettuccine according to package instructions.

2. In your skillet, heat butter in medium heat. Add minced garlic then cook 'til fragrant.

3. Add scallops to your skillet and sear until browned on both sides.

4. Pour in your heavy cream and Parmesan cheese, stirring 'til the sauce thickens. Season using salt and pepper.

5. Toss cooked fettuccine with the creamy garlic Parmesan sauce and scallops. Garnish using chopped parsley.

Per serving: Calories: 480kcal; Fat: 25g; Protein: 30g; Carbs: 35g; Sugar: 2g; Fiber: 2g

Lemon Dill Baked Cod with Couscous

Preparation time: 15 minutes

Cooking time: 20 minutes

Servings: 4

Ingredients:

- 4 cod fillets
- 1 lemon, sliced
- 2 tablespoons olive oil
- 1 tablespoon fresh dill, chopped
- Salt and pepper to taste
- 1 cup couscous, cooked
- Lemon wedges for serving

Directions:

1. Preheat the oven to 375°F.

2. Place cod fillets on your baking sheet. Drizzle using olive oil then season with chopped dill, salt, and pepper.

3. Top each cod fillet with lemon slices.

4. Bake for 15-20 minutes or 'til the cod is flaky then cooked through.

5. Serve the baked cod over cooked couscous with lemon wedges on the side.

Per serving: Calories: 380kcal; Fat: 12g; Protein: 30g; Carbs: 35g; Sugar: 2g; Fiber: 2g

Seafood Paella with Saffron Rice

Preparation time: 30 minutes

Cooking time: 30 minutes

Servings: 6

Ingredients:

- 1 lb large shrimp, peeled and deveined
- 1 lb mussels, cleaned and debearded
- 1 lb squid, cleaned and sliced into rings
- 2 cups Arborio rice
- 4 cups chicken or seafood broth
- 1/2 teaspoon saffron threads
- 1 onion, finely chopped
- 1 bell pepper, diced
- 2 tomatoes, diced
- 4 cloves garlic, minced
- 1 teaspoon smoked paprika
- 1/2 teaspoon turmeric
- Salt and pepper to taste
- 2 tablespoons olive oil
- Lemon wedges for serving

Directions:

1. In your small bowl, steep saffron threads in warm broth.
2. Heat olive oil in your large paella pan or skillet. Add chopped onion and bell pepper, sauté 'til softened.
3. Add minced garlic, diced tomatoes, smoked paprika, turmeric, salt, and pepper. Cook for 2 minutes.
4. Stir in Arborio rice then cook 'til lightly toasted.
5. Pour in saffron-infused broth then simmer. Arrange shrimp, mussels, and squid on top.
6. Cover then simmer for 20-25 minutes or 'til the rice is cooked and the seafood is done.
7. Serve with lemon wedges.

Per serving: Calories: 500kcal; Fat: 10g; Protein: 30g; Carbs: 75g; Sugar: 3g; Fiber: 5g

Cajun Shrimp Pasta

Preparation time: 20 minutes

Cooking time: 20 minutes

Servings: 4

Ingredients:

- 8 oz linguine pasta
- 1 lb large shrimp, peeled and deveined
- 2 tablespoons Cajun seasoning
- 2 tablespoons olive oil
- 1 onion, that is thinly sliced
- 1 bell pepper, that is thinly sliced
- 2 cloves garlic, minced
- 1 cup cherry tomatoes, halved
- 1 cup heavy cream
- Salt and pepper to taste
- Fresh parsley for garnish

Directions:

1. Cook linguine according to package instructions.

2. Toss shrimp with Cajun seasoning.

3. In your skillet, heat olive oil in medium-high heat. Add shrimp then cook 'til pink.

4. Add sliced onion, bell pepper, and minced garlic. Sauté 'til vegetables are tender.

5. Stir in cherry tomatoes and heavy cream. Simmer 'til the sauce thickens.

6. Season using salt and pepper. Toss cooked linguine with the Cajun shrimp mixture.

7. Garnish using fresh parsley before serving.

Per serving: Calories: 520kcal; Fat: 20g; Protein: 30g; Carbs: 55g; Sugar: 5g; Fiber: 4g

Teriyaki Glazed Salmon with Jasmine Rice

Preparation time: 15 minutes

Cooking time: 15 minutes

Servings: 4

Ingredients:

- 4 salmon fillets
- 1/2 cup teriyaki sauce
- 1/4 cup honey
- 2 tablespoons soy sauce
- 1 tablespoon olive oil
- 2 teaspoons minced ginger
- 2 cups cooked jasmine rice
- Green onions for garnish
- Sesame seeds for garnish

Directions:

1. In your bowl, whisk together teriyaki sauce, honey, soy sauce, olive oil, and minced ginger.

2. Marinate salmon fillets in the teriyaki mixture for 10 minutes.

3. Preheat the oven to 400°F.

4. Bake salmon for 12-15 minutes or 'til cooked through.

5. Serve the teriyaki glazed salmon over cooked jasmine rice. Garnish using sliced green onions and sesame seeds.

Per serving: Calories: 450kcal; Fat: 18g; Protein: 30g; Carbs: 45g; Sugar: 15g; Fiber: 2g

Shrimp and Vegetable Skewers with Wild Rice

Preparation time: 20 minutes

Cooking time: 15 minutes

Servings: 4

Ingredients:

- 1 lb large shrimp, peeled and deveined
- 2 bell peppers, cut into chunks
- 1 zucchini, sliced
- 1 red onion, cut into wedges
- 2 tablespoons olive oil
- 1 teaspoon dried oregano
- 1 teaspoon smoked paprika
- Salt and pepper to taste
- 1.5 cups wild rice, cooked
- Lemon wedges for serving

Directions:

1. Preheat the grill.
2. In your bowl, toss shrimp, bell peppers, zucchini, and red onion with salt, olive oil, dried oregano, smoked paprika, and pepper.
3. Thread shrimp and vegetables onto skewers.
4. Grill skewers for 4-5 minutes per side or 'til shrimp are pink and vegetables are tender.
5. Serve over cooked wild rice with lemon wedges on the side.

Per serving: Calories: 420kcal; Fat: 10g; Protein: 30g; Carbs: 60g; Sugar: 4g; Fiber: 8g

Garlic Buttered Lobster Linguine

Preparation time: 20 minutes

Cooking time: 15 minutes

Servings: 4

Ingredients:

- 8 oz linguine pasta
- 2 lobster tails, meat removed and chopped
- 4 tablespoons unsalted butter
- 4 cloves garlic, minced
- 1/4 cup white wine
- Zest and juice of 1 lemon
- Salt and pepper to taste
- Chopped fresh parsley for garnish

Directions:

1. Cook linguine according to package instructions.
2. In your skillet, melt butter in medium heat. Add minced garlic then sauté until fragrant.
3. Add chopped lobster meat to your skillet then cook 'til opaque.
4. Pour in white wine, lemon zest, and lemon juice. Simmer 'til the sauce thickens.
5. Toss cooked linguine with the garlic buttered lobster. Season using salt and pepper.
6. Garnish using chopped fresh parsley before serving.

Per serving: Calories: 480kcal; Fat: 20g; Protein: 25g; Carbs: 55g; Sugar: 2g; Fiber: 3g

Mediterranean Tuna Salad with Orzo

Preparation time: 15 minutes

Cooking time: 10 minutes

Servings: 4

Ingredients:

- 1 cup orzo pasta, cooked
- 2 cans (5 oz each) tuna, drained
- 1 cucumber, diced
- 1 cup cherry tomatoes, halved
- 1/2 cup Kalamata olives, sliced
- 1/4 cup red onion, finely chopped
- 1/4 cup feta cheese, crumbled
- 2 tablespoons olive oil
- 1 tablespoon red wine vinegar
- 1 teaspoon dried oregano
- Salt and pepper to taste
- Fresh parsley for garnish

Directions:

1. In your large bowl, combine cooked orzo, tuna, diced cucumber, cherry tomatoes, sliced Kalamata olives, chopped red onion, and crumbled feta cheese.

2. In your small bowl, whisk together salt, olive oil, red wine vinegar, dried oregano, and pepper.

3. Place dressing over the tuna and orzo mixture, tossing to coat.

4. Garnish using fresh parsley before serving.

Per serving: Calories: 420kcal; Fat: 18g; Protein: 25g; Carbs: 45g; Sugar: 3g; Fiber: 4g

High-Carb Rice, Pasta, and Soup Recipes

Vegetable Fried Rice with Tofu

Preparation time: 15 minutes

Cooking time: 20 minutes

Servings: 4

Ingredients:

- 2 cups cooked jasmine rice, chilled
- 1 cup firm tofu, cubed
- 1 cup mixed vegetables (carrots, peas, corn)
- 2 eggs, beaten
- 3 tablespoons soy sauce
- 1 tablespoon sesame oil
- 1 tablespoon vegetable oil
- 2 green onions, sliced
- Salt and pepper to taste

Directions:

1. In your wok or large skillet, heat vegetable oil in medium-high heat.

2. Add cubed tofu then cook 'til golden brown. Remove from the pan.

3. In the same pan, add mixed vegetables then sauté until tender.

4. Push vegetables to the side, pour beaten eggs into the empty space, and scramble.

5. Add chilled rice, cooked tofu, soy sauce, sesame oil, salt, and pepper. Stir well to combine.

6. Toss in sliced green onions then cook for an additional 2-3 minutes.

Per serving: Calories: 380kcal; Fat: 15g; Protein: 20g; Carbs: 45g; Sugar: 2g; Fiber: 5g

Chicken and Rice Soup

Preparation time: 15 minutes

Cooking time: 30 minutes

Servings: 6

Ingredients:

- 1 lb boneless, skinless chicken breasts, that is cooked and shredded
- 1 cup carrots, diced
- 1 cup celery, diced
- 1 cup onion, finely chopped
- 2 cloves garlic, minced
- 6 cups chicken broth
- 1 cup long-grain white rice, uncooked
- 1 teaspoon dried thyme
- Salt and pepper to taste
- Fresh parsley for garnish

Directions:

1. In your large pot, sauté onions and garlic 'til softened.
2. Add diced carrots, celery, shredded chicken, chicken broth, uncooked rice, dried thyme, salt, and pepper.
3. Boil, then reduce heat then simmer 'til rice is cooked and vegetables are tender.
4. Garnish using fresh parsley before serving.

Per serving: Calories: 320kcal; Fat: 5g; Protein: 25g; Carbs: 45g; Sugar: 2g; Fiber: 3g

Tomato Basil Risotto

Preparation time: 10 minutes

Cooking time: 25 minutes

Servings: 4

Ingredients:

- 1 cup Arborio rice
- 4 cups vegetable broth, heated
- 1 cup cherry tomatoes, halved
- 1/2 cup grated Parmesan cheese
- 1/4 cup fresh basil, chopped
- 1/4 cup white wine
- 1 onion, finely chopped
- 2 tablespoons olive oil
- 2 cloves garlic, minced
- Salt and pepper to taste

Directions:

1. In your large skillet, sauté chopped onions and minced garlic in olive oil until translucent.
2. Add Arborio rice then cook for 2 minutes, stirring constantly.
3. Pour in white wine then cook 'til mostly absorbed.
4. Gradually add hot vegetable broth, one ladle at a time, stirring 'til the liquid is absorbed before adding more.
5. Stir in cherry tomatoes, grated Parmesan cheese, and chopped basil.
6. Season using salt and pepper. Serve warm.

Per serving: Calories: 380kcal; Fat: 12g; Protein: 10g; Carbs: 55g; Sugar: 3g; Fiber: 2g

Lemon Butter Asparagus Risotto

Preparation time: 15 minutes

Cooking time: 25 minutes

Servings: 4

Ingredients:

- 1 cup Arborio rice
- 4 cups vegetable broth, heated
- 1 bunch asparagus, that is trimmed and cut into bite-sized pieces
- 1/2 cup grated Parmesan cheese
- 1/4 cup unsalted butter
- 1/4 cup white wine
- Zest and juice of 1 lemon
- 1 onion, finely chopped
- 2 tablespoons olive oil
- 2 cloves garlic, minced
- Salt and pepper to taste
- Fresh parsley for garnish

Directions:

1. In your large skillet, sauté chopped onions and minced garlic in olive oil until translucent.
2. Add Arborio rice then cook for 2 minutes, stirring constantly.
3. Pour in white wine then cook 'til mostly absorbed.
4. Gradually add hot vegetable broth, one ladle at a time, stirring 'til the liquid is absorbed before adding more.
5. Stir in asparagus, grated Parmesan cheese, lemon zest, and lemon juice.
6. Finish with unsalted butter then season using salt and pepper. Garnish using fresh parsley before serving.

Per serving: Calories: 420kcal; Fat: 18g; Protein: 10g; Carbs: 55g; Sugar: 3g; Fiber: 3g

Chicken Noodle Casserole with Egg Noodles

Preparation time: 20 minutes

Cooking time: 25 minutes

Servings: 6

Ingredients:

- 8 oz egg noodles, cooked
- 2 cups cooked chicken, shredded
- 1 cup frozen peas
- 1 cup carrots, diced
- 1/2 cup mayonnaise
- 1/2 cup sour cream
- 1 cup shredded cheddar cheese
- 1/4 cup grated Parmesan cheese
- 2 tablespoons unsalted butter, melted
- Salt and pepper to taste
- Bread crumbs for topping (optional)

Directions:

1. Preheat the oven to 350°F.
2. In your large bowl, combine cooked egg noodles, shredded chicken, frozen peas, diced carrots, mayonnaise, sour cream, shredded cheddar cheese, grated Parmesan cheese, melted butter, salt, and pepper.
3. Transfer the mixture to your greased baking dish. Top with bread crumbs if desired.
4. Bake for 25 minutes or 'til the casserole is bubbly and golden brown.

Per serving: Calories: 480kcal; Fat: 25g; Protein: 20g; Carbs: 45g; Sugar: 3g; Fiber: 3g

Thai Coconut Curry Noodles with Shrimp

Preparation time: 15 minutes

Cooking time: 20 minutes

Servings: 4

Ingredients:

- 8 oz rice noodles, cooked
- 1 lb shrimp, peeled and deveined
- 1 can (14 oz) coconut milk
- 2 tablespoons red curry paste
- 1 tablespoon soy sauce
- 1 tablespoon fish sauce
- 1 tablespoon brown sugar
- 1 bell pepper, sliced
- 1 carrot, julienned
- 1 zucchini, spiralized
- Fresh cilantro and lime wedges for garnish

Directions:

1. In your large skillet, heat coconut milk in medium heat. Stir in red curry paste, soy sauce, fish sauce, and brown sugar.

2. Add shrimp, bell pepper, julienned carrot, and spiralized zucchini. Simmer until shrimp are pink and vegetables are tender.

3. Toss cooked rice noodles in the coconut curry mixture.

4. Garnish using fresh cilantro then serve with lime wedges.

Per serving: Calories: 480kcal; Fat: 20g; Protein: 25g; Carbs: 55g; Sugar: 6g; Fiber: 3g

Creamy Tomato Basil Pasta with Chickpeas

Preparation time: 15 minutes

Cooking time: 20 minutes

Servings: 4

Ingredients:

- 8 oz penne pasta, cooked
- 1 can (14 oz) diced tomatoes
- 1 can (15 oz) chickpeas, that is drained and rinsed
- 1/2 cup heavy cream
- 1/4 cup grated Parmesan cheese
- 2 tablespoons tomato paste
- 2 tablespoons olive oil
- 2 cloves garlic, minced
- 1 teaspoon dried basil
- Salt and pepper to taste
- Fresh basil for garnish

Directions:

1. In your skillet, sauté minced garlic in olive oil until fragrant.

2. Stir in diced tomatoes, chickpeas, heavy cream, tomato paste, grated Parmesan cheese, dried basil, salt, and pepper.

3. Simmer for 10 minutes, allowing sauce to thicken.

4. Toss the cooked penne pasta in the creamy tomato basil sauce.

5. Garnish using fresh basil before serving.

Per serving: Calories: 480kcal; Fat: 18g; Protein: 15g; Carbs: 65g; Sugar: 5g; Fiber: 6g

Wild Rice and Chicken Casserole

Preparation time: 20 minutes

Cooking time: 40 minutes

Servings: 6

Ingredients:

- 1 cup wild rice, uncooked
- 2 cups cooked chicken, shredded
- 1 cup mushrooms, sliced
- 1 cup broccoli florets
- 1/2 cup carrots, diced
- 1/2 cup celery, diced
- 1/4 cup butter
- 1/4 cup all-purpose flour
- 2 cups chicken broth
- 1 cup milk
- 1 teaspoon dried thyme
- Salt and pepper to taste
- 1 cup shredded cheddar cheese

Directions:

1. Preheat the oven to 375°F.

2. Cook wild rice according to package instructions.

3. In your large skillet, sauté mushrooms, broccoli, carrots, and celery in butter 'til vegetables are tender.

4. Stir in all-purpose flour, then gradually add chicken broth and milk, stirring 'til the sauce thickens.

5. Add cooked wild rice, shredded chicken, dried thyme, salt, and pepper. Mix well.

6. Place the mixture to a greased baking dish. Top with shredded cheddar cheese.

7. Bake for 25-30 minutes or 'til the casserole is bubbly and the cheese is melted.

Per serving: Calories: 420kcal; Fat: 20g; Protein: 25g; Carbs: 35g; Sugar: 4g; Fiber: 4g

Spicy Sausage and Orzo Soup

Preparation time: 15 minutes

Cooking time: 25 minutes

Servings: 6

Ingredients:

- 1 lb spicy sausage, sliced
- 1 cup orzo pasta, uncooked
- 1 onion, diced
- 2 carrots, sliced
- 2 celery stalks, sliced
- 3 cloves garlic, minced
- 6 cups chicken broth
- 1 can (14 oz) diced tomatoes
- 1 teaspoon dried oregano
- 1/2 teaspoon red pepper flakes (optional)
- Salt and pepper to taste
- Fresh parsley for garnish

Directions:

1. In your large pot, brown sliced spicy sausage.

2. Add diced onions, sliced carrots, sliced celery, and minced garlic. Sauté 'til vegetables are softened.

3. Pour in chicken broth, salt, diced tomatoes, orzo pasta, dried oregano, red pepper flakes, and pepper.

4. Simmer until orzo is cooked and flavors are well combined.

5. Garnish using fresh parsley before serving.

Per serving: Calories: 450kcal; Fat: 25g; Protein: 20g; Carbs: 35g; Sugar: 4g; Fiber: 3g

Broccoli and Cheddar Stuffed Baked Potatoes

Preparation time: 10 minutes

Cooking time: 1 hour

Servings: 4

Ingredients:

- 4 large baking potatoes
- 2 cups broccoli florets, steamed
- 1 cup shredded cheddar cheese
- 1/2 cup sour cream
- 2 tablespoons butter
- Salt and pepper to taste
- Chopped chives for garnish

Directions:

1. Preheat the oven to 400°F.

2. Scrub and pierce baking potatoes. Bake for 45-60 minutes or 'til tender.

3. Cut a slit in each baked potato and fluff the insides using a fork.

4. In your bowl, mix steamed broccoli, shredded cheddar cheese, sour cream, butter, salt, and pepper.

5. Stuff each baked potato with the broccoli and cheddar mixture.

6. Garnish using chopped chives before serving.

Per serving: Calories: 380kcal; Fat: 18g; Protein: 15g; Carbs: 45g; Sugar: 2g; Fiber: 5g

Spanish Chickpea and Rice Stew

Preparation time: 15 minutes

Cooking time: 30 minutes

Servings: 6

Ingredients:

- 1 cup long-grain white rice
- 2 cans (15 oz each) chickpeas, that is drained and rinsed
- 1 onion, finely chopped
- 1 bell pepper, diced
- 2 tomatoes, diced
- 3 cloves garlic, minced
- 4 cups vegetable broth
- 1 teaspoon smoked paprika
- 1/2 teaspoon cumin
- 1/2 teaspoon turmeric
- Salt and pepper to taste
- Fresh parsley for garnish

Directions:

1. In your large pot, sauté chopped onions, diced bell peppers, and minced garlic 'til softened.

2. Stir in diced tomatoes, chickpeas, long-grain white rice, smoked paprika, cumin, turmeric, salt, and pepper.

3. Pour in vegetable broth then boil. Reduce heat then simmer 'til rice is cooked and flavors are well combined.

4. Garnish using fresh parsley before serving.

Per serving: Calories: 350kcal; Fat: 2g; Protein: 12g; Carbs: 65g; Sugar: 4g; Fiber: 8g

High-Carb Vegetarian Recipes

Chickpea and Spinach Curry with Basmati Rice

Preparation time: 15 minutes

Cooking time: 25 minutes

Servings: 4

Ingredients:

- 2 cans (15 oz each) chickpeas, that is drained and rinsed
- 1 onion, finely chopped
- 2 tomatoes, diced
- 3 cups fresh spinach
- 1 can (14 oz) coconut milk
- 2 tablespoons curry powder
- 1 tablespoon vegetable oil
- 2 teaspoons minced ginger
- 2 cloves garlic, minced
- Salt and pepper to taste
- Cooked basmati rice for serving

Directions:

1. In your large skillet, sauté chopped onions, minced ginger, and minced garlic in vegetable oil until onions are translucent.

2. Add diced tomatoes then cook 'til softened.

3. Stir in chickpeas, curry powder, coconut milk, fresh spinach, salt, and pepper.

4. Simmer for 15 minutes or 'til the curry thickens.

5. Serve over cooked basmati rice.

Per serving: Calories: 450kcal; Fat: 15g; Protein: 15g; Carbs: 65g; Sugar: 4g; Fiber: 12g

Lentil and Vegetable Stew with Quinoa

Preparation time: 15 minutes

Cooking time: 30 minutes

Servings: 6

Ingredients:

- 1 cup dry green lentils, rinsed
- 1 cup quinoa, rinsed
- 1 onion, diced
- 2 carrots, diced
- 2 celery stalks, diced
- 3 cloves garlic, minced
- 1 can (14 oz) diced tomatoes
- 6 cups vegetable broth
- 2 teaspoons ground cumin
- 1 teaspoon smoked paprika
- Salt and pepper to taste
- Fresh cilantro for garnish

Directions:

1. In your large pot, sauté diced onions, carrots, celery, and minced garlic 'til softened.

2. Add dry lentils, quinoa, diced tomatoes, vegetable broth, ground cumin, smoked paprika, salt, and pepper.

3. Boil, then reduce heat then simmer 'til lentils and quinoa are cooked.

4. Garnish using fresh cilantro before serving.

Per serving: Calories: 350kcal; Fat: 2g; Protein: 18g; Carbs: 65g; Sugar: 4g; Fiber: 12g

Eggplant Parmesan with Whole Wheat Pasta

Preparation time: 20 minutes

Cooking time: 30 minutes

Servings: 4

Ingredients:

- 1 large eggplant, sliced
- 2 cups whole wheat pasta, cooked
- 1 cup marinara sauce
- 1 cup shredded mozzarella cheese
- 1/2 cup grated Parmesan cheese
- 2 tablespoons olive oil
- 2 teaspoons dried oregano
- Salt and pepper to taste
- Fresh basil for garnish

Directions:

1. Preheat the oven to 375°F.

2. Brush eggplant slices with olive oil then season using salt, pepper, and dried oregano.

3. Bake eggplant slices for 15 minutes or 'til tender.

4. In your baking dish, layer cooked whole wheat pasta, marinara sauce, baked eggplant slices, shredded mozzarella cheese, and grated Parmesan cheese.

5. Repeat layers, finish with a layer of cheese on top.

6. Bake for 15-20 minutes or 'til the cheese is melted and bubbly.

7. Garnish using fresh basil before serving.

Per serving: Calories: 420kcal; Fat: 18g; Protein: 15g; Carbs: 55g; Sugar: 6g; Fiber: 10g

Sweet Potato and Black Bean Burritos

Preparation time: 20 minutes

Cooking time: 30 minutes

Servings: 4

Ingredients:

- 2 large sweet potatoes, peeled and diced
- 1 can (15 oz) black beans, that is drained and rinsed
- 1 cup corn kernels
- 1 bell pepper, diced
- 1 onion, finely chopped
- 2 teaspoons ground cumin
- 1 teaspoon chili powder
- 1/2 teaspoon smoked paprika
- 4 large whole wheat tortillas
- 1 cup salsa
- 1 cup shredded cheddar cheese
- Fresh cilantro for garnish

Directions:

1. Boil or steam diced sweet potatoes until tender. Mash them in a bowl.
2. In your skillet, sauté chopped onions and diced bell peppers 'til softened.
3. Add mashed sweet potatoes, black beans, corn kernels, ground cumin, chili powder, and smoked paprika. Mix well.
4. Warm whole wheat tortillas and spoon sweet potato and black bean mixture onto each tortilla.
5. Top with salsa and shredded cheddar cheese. Roll into burritos.
6. Bake in the oven for 10 minutes or 'til the cheese is melted.
7. Garnish using fresh cilantro before serving.

Per serving: Calories: 380kcal; Fat: 10g; Protein: 15g; Carbs: 60g; Sugar: 8g; Fiber: 12g

Lentil and Vegetable Stir-Fry with Brown Rice

Preparation time: 15 minutes

Cooking time: 25 minutes

Servings: 4

Ingredients:

- 1 cup dry brown lentils, rinsed
- 2 cups cooked brown rice
- 1 bell pepper, sliced
- 1 zucchini, sliced
- 1 carrot, julienned
- 1 cup broccoli florets
- 2 tablespoons soy sauce
- 1 tablespoon sesame oil
- 1 tablespoon vegetable oil
- 2 teaspoons minced ginger
- 2 cloves garlic, minced
- Green onions for garnish

Directions:

1. Cook brown lentils according to package instructions.

2. In your wok or large skillet, heat vegetable oil in medium-high heat.

3. Add sliced bell peppers, zucchini, julienned carrots, and broccoli florets. Stir-fry 'til vegetables are crisp-tender.

4. Push vegetables to the side, add minced ginger and minced garlic to the empty space, then sauté until fragrant.

5. Stir in cooked brown lentils, cooked brown rice, soy sauce, and sesame oil. Mix well.

6. Cook for an additional 3-5 minutes or 'til everything is heated through.

7. Garnish using sliced green onions before serving.

Per serving: Calories: 400kcal; Fat: 10g; Protein: 18g; Carbs: 65g; Sugar: 4g; Fiber: 10g

Butternut Squash and Sage Risotto

Preparation time: 15 minutes

Cooking time: 30 minutes

Servings: 4

Ingredients:

- 1 cup Arborio rice
- 2 cups butternut squash, diced
- 1/2 cup white wine
- 1 onion, finely chopped
- 4 cups vegetable broth, heated
- 1/2 cup Parmesan cheese, grated
- 2 tablespoons olive oil
- 1 tablespoon fresh sage, chopped
- Salt and pepper to taste

Directions:

1. In your large skillet, sauté chopped onions in olive oil until translucent.

2. Add Arborio rice then cook for 2 minutes, stirring constantly.

3. Pour in white wine then cook 'til mostly absorbed.

4. Gradually add hot vegetable broth, one ladle at a time, stirring 'til the liquid is absorbed before adding more.

5. Stir in diced butternut squash and continue cooking until rice is creamy and squash is tender.

6. Finish with grated Parmesan cheese, chopped fresh sage, salt, and pepper.

Per serving: Calories: 420kcal; Fat: 10g; Protein: 10g; Carbs: 75g; Sugar: 4g; Fiber: 6g

Spinach and Ricotta Stuffed Shells

Preparation time: 20 minutes

Cooking time: 30 minutes

Servings: 4

Ingredients:

- 16 jumbo pasta shells, cooked
- 2 cups ricotta cheese
- 2 cups fresh spinach, chopped
- 1 cup mozzarella cheese, shredded
- 1/2 cup Parmesan cheese, grated
- 2 cloves garlic, minced
- 1 egg
- 2 cups marinara sauce
- 1 tablespoon olive oil
- Salt and pepper to taste
- Fresh basil for garnish

Directions:

1. Preheat the oven to 375°F.

2. In your bowl, combine ricotta cheese, chopped spinach, mozzarella cheese, grated Parmesan cheese, minced garlic, egg, salt, and pepper.

3. Stuff each cooked pasta shell using the spinach and ricotta mixture.

4. In your baking dish, spread olive oil and a thin layer of marinara sauce.

5. Arrange the stuffed shells in your baking dish and cover with the remaining marinara sauce.

6. Bake for 25-30 minutes or 'til the cheese is melted and bubbly.

7. Garnish using fresh basil before serving.

Per serving: Calories: 480kcal; Fat: 20g; Protein: 25g; Carbs: 55g; Sugar: 6g; Fiber: 5g

Quinoa and Black Bean Salad

Preparation time: 15 minutes

Cooking time: 15 minutes

Servings: 4

Ingredients:

- 1 cup quinoa, cooked
- 1 can (15 oz) black beans, that is drained and rinsed
- 1 cup corn kernels
- 1 bell pepper, diced
- 1/2 red onion, finely chopped
- 1/4 cup cilantro, chopped
- 2 tablespoons olive oil
- 1 lime, juiced
- 1 teaspoon ground cumin
- Salt and pepper to taste
- Avocado slices for garnish

Directions:

1. In your large bowl, combine cooked quinoa, black beans, corn kernels, diced bell pepper, finely chopped red onion, and chopped cilantro.

2. In your small bowl, whisk together olive oil, lime juice, ground cumin, salt, and pepper.

3. Place dressing over the quinoa mixture then toss to combine.

4. Garnish using avocado slices before serving.

Per serving: Calories: 380kcal; Fat: 12g; Protein: 12g; Carbs: 55g; Sugar: 3g; Fiber: 10g

Mediterranean Couscous Salad

Preparation time: 15 minutes

Cooking time: 5 minutes

Servings: 4

Ingredients:

- 1 cup couscous, cooked
- 1 cucumber, diced
- 1 cup cherry tomatoes, halved
- 1/2 cup Kalamata olives, sliced
- 1/4 cup red onion, finely chopped
- 1/4 cup feta cheese, crumbled
- 2 tablespoons olive oil
- 1 tablespoon red wine vinegar
- 1 teaspoon dried oregano
- Salt and pepper to taste
- Fresh parsley for garnish

Directions:

1. In your large bowl, combine cooked couscous, diced cucumber, halved cherry tomatoes, sliced Kalamata olives, finely chopped red onion, and crumbled feta cheese.

2. In your small bowl, whisk together salt, olive oil, red wine vinegar, dried oregano, and pepper.

3. Place dressing over the couscous mixture then toss to combine.

4. Garnish using fresh parsley before serving.

Per serving: Calories: 350kcal; Fat: 15g; Protein: 10g; Carbs: 45g; Sugar: 4g; Fiber: 6g

Roasted Vegetable and Hummus Wrap

Preparation time: 15 minutes

Cooking time: 20 minutes

Servings: 2

Ingredients:

- 2 large whole wheat wraps
- 1 cup hummus
- 2 cups mixed vegetables (bell peppers, zucchini, cherry tomatoes), sliced
- 2 tablespoons olive oil
- 1 teaspoon dried oregano
- Salt and pepper to taste
- Fresh spinach leaves for filling

Directions:

1. Preheat the oven to 400°F.

2. Toss sliced vegetables with olive oil, dried oregano, salt, and pepper.

3. Roast the vegetables in to your oven for 15-20 minutes or 'til they are tender and slightly caramelized.

4. Spread hummus on each whole wheat wrap.

5. Place a handful of your fresh spinach leaves on each wrap and top with the roasted vegetables.

6. Roll the wraps and cut them in half before serving.

Per serving: Calories: 450kcal; Fat: 25g; Protein: 15g; Carbs: 50g; Sugar: 4g; Fiber: 10g

Pumpkin and Sage Pasta with Parmesan

Preparation time: 20 minutes

Cooking time: 15 minutes

Servings: 4

Ingredients:

- 8 oz whole wheat pasta, cooked
- 1 can (15 oz) pumpkin puree
- 1/2 cup vegetable broth
- 1/4 cup Parmesan cheese, grated
- 2 tablespoons olive oil
- 1 tablespoon fresh sage, chopped
- 2 cloves garlic, minced
- Salt and pepper to taste
- Pine nuts for garnish

Directions:

1. In your saucepan, heat olive oil in medium heat. Add minced garlic and chopped fresh sage, sautéing until fragrant.

2. Stir in pumpkin puree and vegetable broth, allowing the mixture to simmer for 5 minutes.

3. Add cooked whole wheat pasta to the pumpkin sauce, tossing 'til the pasta is well coated.

4. Stir in your grated Parmesan cheese, salt, and pepper.

5. Garnish using pine nuts before serving.

Per serving: Calories: 380kcal; Fat: 15g; Protein: 10g; Carbs: 50g; Sugar: 4g; Fiber: 8g

High-Carb Dessert Recipes

Mixed Berry Crisp with Oat Topping

Preparation time: 15 minutes

Cooking time: 35 minutes

Servings: 6

Ingredients:

- 4 cups mixed berries (strawberries, blueberries, raspberries)
- 1/4 cup granulated sugar
- 1 tablespoon cornstarch
- 1 cup old-fashioned oats
- 1/2 cup whole wheat flour
- 1/3 cup brown sugar
- 1/4 cup melted butter
- 1 teaspoon cinnamon
- Pinch of salt
- Vanilla ice cream for serving (optional)

Directions:

1. Preheat the oven to 350°F.

2. In your bowl, toss mixed berries with granulated sugar and cornstarch. Transfer to a baking dish.

3. In another bowl, combine old-fashioned oats, whole wheat flour, brown sugar, melted butter, cinnamon, and a pinch of salt. Mix until crumbly.

4. Sprinkle the oat topping over the berries.

5. Bake for 35 minutes or 'til the topping is golden brown then the berries are bubbling.

6. Allow to cool slightly before serving. Top with vanilla ice cream if desired.

Per serving: Calories: 280kcal; Fat: 10g; Protein: 4g; Carbs: 45g; Sugar: 20g; Fiber: 7g

Chocolate Chip Banana Bread

Preparation time: 15 minutes

Cooking time: 1 hour

Servings: 10

Ingredients:

- 3 ripe bananas, mashed
- 1/2 cup unsalted butter, melted
- 1/2 cup granulated sugar
- 2 large eggs
- 1 teaspoon vanilla extract
- 1 3/4 cups all-purpose flour
- 1 teaspoon baking soda
- 1/4 teaspoon salt
- 1 cup chocolate chips

Directions:

1. Preheat the oven to 350°F. Grease a loaf pan.

2. In your large bowl, mix mashed bananas, melted butter, granulated sugar, eggs, and vanilla extract.

3. In your separate bowl, whisk together all-purpose flour, baking soda, and salt.

4. Combine your wet and dry ingredients 'til just incorporated.

5. Fold in the chocolate chips.

6. Pour batter in to your prepared loaf pan then bake for 1 hour or 'til a toothpick inserted comes out clean.

7. Let the banana bread to cool before slicing.

Per serving: Calories: 320kcal; Fat: 14g; Protein: 4g; Carbs: 46g; Sugar: 24g; Fiber: 3g

Lemon Blueberry Muffins

Preparation time: 15 minutes

Cooking time: 20 minutes

Servings: 12

Ingredients:

- 2 cups whole wheat flour
- 1/2 cup granulated sugar
- 1 tablespoon baking powder
- 1/4 teaspoon salt
- 1 cup milk
- 1/3 cup vegetable oil
- 1 large egg
- 1 teaspoon vanilla extract
- Zest of 1 lemon
- 1 1/2 cups of fresh or frozen blueberries

Directions:

1. Preheat the oven to 400°F. Line a muffin tin using paper liners.

2. In your large bowl, whisk together whole wheat flour, granulated sugar, baking powder, and salt.

3. In another bowl, mix together milk, vegetable oil, egg, vanilla extract, and lemon zest.

4. Place the wet ingredients to the dry ingredients, stirring until just combined.

5. Gently fold in the blueberries.

6. Spoon batter into your muffin cups, filling each about two-thirds full.

7. Bake for 18-20 minutes or 'til a toothpick inserted comes out clean.

8. Let the muffins to cool in the tin for 5 minutes before transferring to your wire rack.

Per serving: Calories: 180kcal; Fat: 7g; Protein: 3g; Carbs: 28g; Sugar: 10g; Fiber: 3g

Classic Rice Pudding with Raisins

Preparation time: 10 minutes

Cooking time: 45 minutes

Servings: 6

Ingredients:

- 1 cup Arborio rice
- 4 cups whole milk
- 1/2 cup granulated sugar
- 1/2 cup raisins
- 1 teaspoon vanilla extract
- 1/2 teaspoon ground cinnamon
- Pinch of salt
- Ground nutmeg for garnish

Directions:

1. In your medium saucepan, combine Arborio rice, whole milk, granulated sugar, raisins, vanilla extract, ground cinnamon, and a pinch of salt.

2. Bring the mixture to a simmer in medium heat, stirring frequently.

3. Lower heat to low, simmer, stirring occasionally, for 30-40 minutes or 'til the rice is tender and the pudding has thickened.

4. Remove from heat then let it cool slightly before serving.

5. Sprinkle ground nutmeg on top for garnish.

Per serving: Calories: 300kcal; Fat: 5g; Protein: 7g; Carbs: 55g; Sugar: 20g; Fiber: 1g

Cherry Almond Clafoutis

Preparation time: 15 minutes

Cooking time: 40 minutes

Servings: 8

Ingredients:

- 2 cups fresh or frozen cherries, pitted
- 1/2 cup almond flour
- 1/2 cup all-purpose flour
- 1/2 cup granulated sugar
- 3 large eggs
- 1 1/2 cups whole milk
- 1 teaspoon almond extract
- 1/2 teaspoon vanilla extract
- Powdered sugar for dusting

Directions:

1. Preheat the oven to 350°F. Grease a baking dish.

2. Arrange the pitted cherries in the baking dish.

3. In your bowl, whisk together almond flour, all-purpose flour, granulated sugar, eggs, whole milk, almond extract, and vanilla extract 'til smooth.

4. Pour batter over the cherries in the baking dish.

5. Bake for 35-40 minutes or 'til the clafoutis is set and golden brown.

6. Let it cool slightly before dusting using powdered sugar.

Per serving: Calories: 220kcal; Fat: 8g; Protein: 7g; Carbs: 30g; Sugar: 18g; Fiber: 2g

Pumpkin Pie with Whipped Cream

Preparation time: 20 minutes

Cooking time: 50 minutes

Servings: 8

Ingredients:

- 1 pie crust (store-bought or homemade)
- 1 can (15 oz) pumpkin puree
- 1 cup evaporated milk
- 2 large eggs
- 3/4 cup granulated sugar
- 1 teaspoon ground cinnamon
- 1/2 teaspoon ground ginger
- 1/4 teaspoon ground cloves
- 1/2 teaspoon salt
- Whipped cream for topping

Directions:

1. Preheat the oven to 425°F.
2. In your bowl, whisk together pumpkin puree, evaporated milk, eggs, granulated sugar, ground cinnamon, ground ginger, ground cloves, and salt until well combined.
3. Roll out the pie crust then fit it into a pie dish.
4. Pour pumpkin mixture into the pie crust.
5. Bake for 15 minutes, then lower your oven temperature to 350 deg. F then continue baking for 35-40 minutes or 'til a toothpick inserted comes out clean.
6. Let the pie to cool before serving. Top with whipped cream.

Per serving: Calories: 320kcal; Fat: 15g; Protein: 6g; Carbs: 42g; Sugar: 20g; Fiber: 2g

Orange Glazed Pound Cake

Preparation time: 20 minutes

Cooking time: 50 minutes

Servings: 10

Ingredients:

- 2 cups all-purpose flour
- 1 cup unsalted butter, softened
- 1 cup granulated sugar
- 4 large eggs
- 1/2 cup sour cream
- 1/4 cup orange juice
- Zest of 2 oranges
- 1 teaspoon vanilla extract
- 1 teaspoon baking powder
- 1/2 teaspoon salt
- Powdered sugar for garnish

Directions:

1. Preheat the oven to 325°F. Grease and flour a loaf pan.
2. In your bowl, whisk together all-purpose flour, baking powder, and salt.
3. In another bowl, cream together your softened butter and granulated sugar until light and fluffy.
4. Place eggs one at a time, beating well after each addition. Stir in vanilla extract.
5. Gradually place the dry ingredients to the wet ingredients, alternating with sour cream and orange juice. Mix until just combined.
6. Fold in the orange zest.
7. Pour batter in to your prepared loaf pan and smooth the top.
8. Bake for 45-50 minutes or 'til a toothpick inserted comes out clean.
9. Let the pound cake to cool in the pan for 10 minutes before transferring to your wire rack.
10. Dust with powdered sugar before serving.

Per serving: Calories: 380kcal; Fat: 20g; Protein: 5g; Carbs: 45g; Sugar: 20g; Fiber: 1g

Caramelized Banana Splits

Preparation time: 10 minutes

Cooking time: 5 minutes

Servings: 4

Ingredients:

- 4 ripe bananas, peeled and halved
- 1/4 cup unsalted butter
- 1/4 cup brown sugar
- 1 teaspoon vanilla extract
- Vanilla ice cream
- Whipped cream
- Chopped nuts for garnish

Directions:

1. In your skillet, melt butter in medium heat.

2. Add brown sugar and vanilla extract, stirring 'til the sugar is dissolved.

3. Place banana halves in the skillet then cook for 2-3 minutes on each side, until caramelized.

4. Remove bananas from the skillet and place two halves in each serving dish.

5. Top with a scoop of your vanilla ice cream, whipped cream, then garnish with chopped nuts.

Per serving: Calories: 320kcal; Fat: 15g; Protein: 3g; Carbs: 45g; Sugar: 30g; Fiber: 3g

High-Carb Snack and Drink Recipes

Trail Mix with Dried Fruits and Nuts

Preparation time: 5 minutes

Cooking time: 0 minutes

Servings: 4

Ingredients:

- 1 cup mixed nuts (almonds, walnuts, cashews)
- 1/2 cup dried cranberries
- 1/2 cup raisins
- 1/4 cup dark chocolate chips
- 1/4 cup banana chips

Directions:

1. In your bowl, mix together mixed nuts, dried cranberries, raisins, dark chocolate chips, and banana chips.

2. Toss until well combined.

3. Divide into 1/4-cup servings for a quick and convenient snack.

Per serving: Calories: 250kcal; Fat: 15g; Protein: 5g; Carbs: 28g; Sugar: 15g; Fiber: 4g

Roasted Chickpeas with Paprika

Preparation time: 10 minutes

Cooking time: 30 minutes

Servings: 4

Ingredients:

- 2 cans (15 oz each) chickpeas, that is drained and rinsed
- 2 tablespoons olive oil
- 1 teaspoon smoked paprika
- 1/2 teaspoon garlic powder
- 1/2 teaspoon cumin
- Salt to taste

Directions:

1. Preheat the oven to 400°F.
2. Pat chickpeas dry using a paper towel then spread them on your baking sheet.
3. In your bowl, mix together olive oil, smoked paprika, garlic powder, cumin, and salt.
4. Drizzle the spice mixture over the chickpeas then toss to coat.
5. Roast in to your oven for 30 minutes, shaking the pan occasionally, 'til the chickpeas are crispy.
6. Allow to cool before serving.

Per serving: Calories: 220kcal; Fat: 7g; Protein: 9g; Carbs: 32g; Sugar: 5g; Fiber: 8g

Fruit Smoothie with Spinach and Berries

Preparation time: 5 minutes

Cooking time: 0 minutes

Servings: 2

Ingredients:

- 1 cup spinach leaves
- 1 cup mixed berries (strawberries, blueberries, raspberries)
- 1 banana, peeled
- 1 cup plain yogurt
- 1/2 cup orange juice
- Ice cubes (optional)

Directions:

1. In your blender, combine spinach leaves, mixed berries, banana, plain yogurt, and orange juice.
2. Blend 'til smooth.
3. Add ice cubes if desired then blend again.
4. Pour into glasses and enjoy.

Per serving: Calories: 180kcal; Fat: 2g; Protein: 7g; Carbs: 40g; Sugar: 25g; Fiber: 6g

Peanut Butter and Banana Sandwich

Preparation time: 5 minutes

Cooking time: 0 minutes

Servings: 1

Ingredients:

- 2 slices whole wheat bread
- 2 tablespoons peanut butter
- 1 banana, sliced

Directions:

1. Spread your peanut butter evenly on one side of each bread slice.
2. Place banana slices on one of the bread slices.
3. Top with the other bread slice, peanut butter side down.
4. Press gently and cut in half if desired.

Per serving: Calories: 380kcal; Fat: 18g; Protein: 10g; Carbs: 50g; Sugar: 18g; Fiber: 8g

Blueberry Almond Rice Cakes

Preparation time: 5 minutes

Cooking time: 0 minutes

Servings: 2

Ingredients:

- 2 rice cakes
- 4 tablespoons almond butter
- 1/2 cup fresh blueberries
- Drizzle of honey

Directions:

1. Spread almond butter evenly on each rice cake.
2. Top with fresh blueberries.
3. Drizzle using honey before serving.

Per serving: Calories: 300kcal; Fat: 16g; Protein: 8g; Carbs: 34g; Sugar: 14g; Fiber: 4g

Apple Slices with Caramel Dip

Preparation time: 10 minutes

Cooking time: 0 minutes

Servings: 2

Ingredients:

- 2 apples, sliced
- 1/4 cup caramel dip (store-bought or homemade)

Directions:

1. Arrange apple slices on a plate.
2. Serve with a side of caramel dip for dipping.

Per serving: Calories: 180kcal; Fat: 2g; Protein: 1g; Carbs: 45g; Sugar: 35g; Fiber: 5g

Cottage Cheese with Pineapple

Preparation time: 5 minutes

Cooking time: 0 minutes

Servings: 2

Ingredients:

- 1 cup cottage cheese
- 1 cup fresh pineapple chunks

Directions:

1. In your bowl, combine cottage cheese and fresh pineapple chunks.

2. Mix well then serve.

Per serving: Calories: 220kcal; Fat: 5g; Protein: 16g; Carbs: 30g; Sugar: 20g; Fiber: 3g

Raspberry Lemonade with Fresh Mint

Preparation time: 10 minutes

Cooking time: 0 minutes

Servings: 4

Ingredients:

- 2 cups fresh raspberries
- 1 cup freshly squeezed lemon juice
- 1/2 cup honey or agave nectar
- 6 cups cold water
- Fresh mint leaves for garnish
- Ice cubes

Directions:

1. In your blender, puree fresh raspberries.

2. Strain the raspberry puree to remove seeds, collecting the raspberry juice.

3. In your pitcher, combine raspberry juice, freshly squeezed lemon juice, honey or agave nectar, and cold water. Stir well.

4. Refrigerate until chilled.

5. Serve over ice cubes then garnish with fresh mint leaves.

Per serving: Calories: 80kcal; Fat: 0g; Protein: 1g; Carbs: 21g; Sugar: 17g; Fiber: 5g

Chapter 9: 30-Day Meal Plan

Day	Breakfast	Lunch	Dinner	Dessert	Carb Cycling
1	Apple Cinnamon Quinoa Porridge	Orange Glazed Chicken with Sweet Potatoes	Lentil and Vegetable Stew with Quinoa	Chocolate Chip Banana Bread	High
2	Zucchini and Cheese Muffins	Grilled Lemon Garlic Chicken	Creamy Tomato Basil Zoodle Soup	Berry and Cream Cheese Fat Bombs	Low
3	Peanut Butter Banana Breakfast Wrap	Tomato Basil Risotto	Teriyaki Chicken Skewers with Jasmine Rice	Orange Glazed Pound Cake	High
4	Broccoli and Cheddar Breakfast Muffins	Shrimp and Avocado Salad	Beef and Vegetable Stir-Fry	Chocolate Peanut Butter Fat Bombs	Low
5	Berry and Yogurt Parfait	Tuna and Brown Rice Casserole	Vegetable Fried Rice with Tofu	Classic Rice Pudding with Raisins	High
6	Cauliflower Hash Browns	Low-Carb Chicken and Vegetable Stir-Fry	Coconut Lime Grilled Mahi-Mahi	Keto Cheesecake Bites	Low
7	Classic Oatmeal with Fresh Fruits	Lemon Herb Chicken with Roasted Potatoes	Grilled Tilapia Tacos with Mango Salsa	Mixed Berry Crisp with Oat Topping	High
8	Spinach and Feta Omelet	Lemon Herb Grilled Steak	Spinach and Sausage Soup	Dark Chocolate and Almond Bark	Low
9	Tropical Fruit Salad with Honey Drizzle	Creamy Tomato Basil Pasta with Chickpeas	Chili Lime Grilled Chicken Tacos	Caramelized Banana Splits	High
10	Smoked Salmon and Cream Cheese Roll-Ups	Spicy Cilantro Lime Tilapia	Italian Sausage and Peppers	Keto Chocolate Avocado Mousse	Low
11	Sweet Potato Hash with Eggs	Creamy Garlic Parmesan Pasta with Scallops	Thai Coconut Curry Noodles with Shrimp	Lemon Blueberry Muffins	High
12	Avocado and Bacon Egg Cups	Broccoli and Cheese Soup	Zucchini Noodles with Pesto and Shrimp	Vanilla Coconut Flour Mug Cake	Low
13	Whole Grain Pancakes with Maple Syrup	Sweet and Sour Meatballs with Quinoa	Lemon Garlic Butter Shrimp with Linguine	Pumpkin Pie with Whipped Cream	High
14	Keto Egg Salad Lettuce Wraps	Chicken and Broccoli Casserole	Spaghetti Squash with Meat Sauce	Almond Flour Chocolate Chip Cookies	Low

15	Brown Sugar and Cinnamon French Toast	Broccoli and Cheddar Stuffed Baked Potatoes	Balsamic Glazed Beef with Pasta	Cherry Almond Clafoutis	High
16	Keto Chia Seed Pudding	Garlic Butter Scallops	Shirataki Noodles with Alfredo Sauce	Coconut Flour Lemon Poppy Seed Muffins	Low
17	Blueberry Almond Butter Smoothie Bowl	Shrimp and Vegetable Skewers with Wild Rice	Chicken and Rice Soup	Classic Rice Pudding with Raisins	High
18	Turkey and Veggie Breakfast Skillet	Crispy Baked Chicken Thighs	Baked Turkey Meatballs with Zucchini	Avocado Chocolate Pudding	Low
19	Peanut Butter Banana Breakfast Wrap	Beef and Broccoli with Noodles	Teriyaki Glazed Salmon with Jasmine Rice	Caramelized Banana Splits	High
20	Almond Flour Pancakes	Creamy Cauliflower and Bacon Soup	Grilled Garlic Butter Shrimp Skewers	Almond Flour Blueberry Muffins	Low
21	Classic Oatmeal with Fresh Fruits	Chicken Noodle Casserole with Egg Noodles	Beef and Vegetable Stir-Fry with Brown Rice	Chocolate Chip Banana Bread	High
22	Broccoli and Cheddar Breakfast Muffins	Cauliflower Fried Rice	Lemon Garlic Butter Baked Salmon	Raspberry Coconut Chia Seed Pudding	Low
23	Apple Cinnamon Quinoa Porridge	Seafood Paella with Saffron Rice	Spanish Chickpea and Rice Stew	Pumpkin Pie with Whipped Cream	High
24	Keto Egg Salad Lettuce Wraps	Pork Tenderloin with Dijon Mustard Glaze	Cucumber and Avocado Salad	Avocado Chocolate Pudding	Low
25	Sweet Potato Hash with Eggs	Pork and Pineapple Skewers with Coconut Rice	Coconut Curry Shrimp with Basmati Rice	Lemon Blueberry Muffins	High
26	Zucchini and Cheese Muffins	Baked Cod with Herbs and Lemon	Cabbage and Beef Skillet	Almond Flour Blueberry Muffins	Low
27	Whole Grain Pancakes with Maple Syrup	Wild Rice and Chicken Casserole	BBQ Pulled Pork Sandwiches	Cherry Almond Clafoutis	High
28	Avocado and Bacon Egg Cups	Mexican Cauliflower Rice	Smoked Salmon Cucumber Bites	Berry and Cream Cheese Fat Bombs	Low
29	Tropical Fruit Salad with Honey Drizzle	Mediterranean Tuna Salad with Orzo	Lemon Butter Asparagus Risotto	Orange Glazed Pound Cake	High
30	Spinach and Feta Omelet	Rosemary Roasted Pork Loin	Spicy Ground Turkey Lettuce Wraps	Vanilla Coconut Flour Mug Cake	Low

Chapter 10:
Conversion Table

Volume Equivalents (Liquid)

US Standard	US Standard (ounces)	Metric (approximate)
2 tablespoons	1 fl. oz.	30 mL
¼ cup	2 fl. oz.	60 mL
½ cup	4 fl. oz.	120 mL
1 cup	8 fl. oz.	240 mL
1½ cups	12 fl. oz.	355 mL
2 cups or 1 pint	16 fl. oz.	475 mL
4 cups or 1 quart	32 fl. oz.	1 L
1 gallon	128 fl. oz.	4 L

Volume Equivalents (Dry)

US Standard	Metric (approximate)
⅛ teaspoon	0.5 mL
¼ teaspoon	1 mL
½ teaspoon	2 mL
¾ teaspoon	4 mL
1 teaspoon	5 mL
1 tablespoon	15 mL
¼ cup	59 mL
⅓ cup	79 mL

½ cup	118 mL
⅔ cup	156 mL
¾ cup	177 mL
1 cup	235 mL
2 cups or 1 pint	475 mL
3 cups	700 mL
4 cups or 1 quart	1 L

Oven Temperatures

Fahrenheit (F)	Celsius (C) (approximate)
250°F	120°C
300°F	150°C
325°F	165°C
350°F	180°C
375°F	190°C
400°F	200°C
425°F	220°C
450°F	230°C

Weight Equivalents

US Standard	Metric (approximate)
1 tablespoon	15 g
½ ounce	15 g
1 ounce	30 g
2 ounces	60 g
4 ounces	115 g
8 ounces	225 g
12 ounces	340 g
16 ounces or 1 pound	455 g

Chapter 11: The Dirty Dozen™ and The Clean Fifteen™

Annually, the Environmental Working Group (EWG) scrutinizes the latest USDA data to create its well-known Clean 15 and Dirty Dozen compilations, categorizing fruits and vegetables based on their pesticide levels. These lists serve as valuable references to inform your produce purchasing decisions, especially if you're on a budget. The Dirty Dozen and Clean 15 can help direct you toward organic options for health reasons, though considerations for environmental and workers' rights also support choosing organic when possible.

The Dirty Dozen™

The 2023 Dirty Dozen list results from the EWG's analysis of USDA data on 46,569 samples of the 46 most popular fruits and vegetables. After the USDA washed and peeled the samples as one would at home, the report revealed that nearly 75% of non-organic fresh produce in the U.S. contained pesticide residues. The EWG scores each type of produce based on various factors, such as the percentage of samples with detectable pesticides, the average number of pesticides found, and the total number of pesticides found on the crop.

Here is the most recent list:

1. Strawberries
2. Spinach
3. Kale, collard, and mustard greens
4. Peaches
5. Pears
6. Nectarines
7. Apples
8. Grapes
9. Bell & Hot Peppers
10. Cherries
11. Blueberries
12. Green Beans

The 2023 Dirty Dozen includes familiar items such as strawberries, spinach, and apples, with blueberries and green beans as new additions. The list doesn't definitively declare which crops pose the highest human health risk but rather highlights those treated with the highest volume and variety of pesticides.

The Clean Fifteen™

The 2023 Clean 15, showcasing produce with lower pesticide levels, features items like avocados and sweet corn. Notably, produce with tough outer peels, husks, or shells tends to rank as the "cleanest."

1. Avocados
2. Sweet corn
3. Pineapple
4. Onions
5. Papaya
6. Sweet peas (frozen)
7. Asparagus
8. Honeydew melon
9. Kiwi
10. Cabbage
11. Mushrooms
12. Mangoes
13. Sweet Potatoes
14. Watermelon
15. Carrots

Carrots are new additions to the Clean 15 list, surpassing cantaloupe for having the fewest detectable pesticide residues. Avocados and sweet corn samples emerged as the cleanest, with less than 2% showing any detectable pesticides. The report emphasizes that approximately 65% of fruit and vegetable samples on this list had no detectable pesticide residues after preparation.

Conclusion

In concluding our journey through the world of Carb Cycling for Beginners, it's evident that this revolutionary approach to nutrition isn't just a diet – it's a lifestyle transformation. As you've delved into the science behind strategic carbohydrate intake and explored the delectable recipes designed for both low-carb and high-carb days, you've equipped yourself with the tools to achieve not only your fitness goals but also a sustained sense of well-being.

Carb Cycling isn't about rigid restrictions or deprivation; it's about empowerment and flexibility. It's an acknowledgment that our bodies are dynamic, and our nutritional needs vary. By embracing this approach, you're not just reshaping your physique; you're redefining your relationship with food. You're learning to appreciate the richness of flavors, the nourishing power of ingredients, and the joy that comes with a well-balanced, sustainable lifestyle.

As you move forward, remember that Carb Cycling isn't a one-size-fits-all solution. It's a customizable, adaptable strategy that evolves with your progress and personal preferences. You've learned to listen to your body, to understand its signals, and to respond with the nourishment it deserves. In doing so, you're not just achieving a healthier weight or enhancing your physical performance – you're nurturing a healthier, more vibrant version of yourself.

Meal planning and preparation have become more than just tasks; they're opportunities to express your creativity in the kitchen, crafting meals that delight your palate while aligning with your fitness goals. You've discovered that achieving a balance between low-carb and high-carb days isn't a challenge but an adventure, a journey filled with delicious discoveries and newfound culinary pleasures.

As you embrace this healthier lifestyle, know that challenges may arise. Cravings, social situations, and the ebb and flow of life can test your commitment. But armed with the knowledge and strategies provided in this guide, you're well-equipped to overcome these obstacles. Your journey is not a linear path; it's a continuous cycle of growth, self-discovery, and transformation.

In the end, Carb Cycling for Beginners isn't just about achieving short-term results; it's about cultivating lasting habits that contribute to a lifelong sense of vitality and well-being. You're not just managing your weight; you're mastering the art of nourishing your body and soul. So, here's to your continued success, to the joy of balanced living, and to the exciting chapters that lie ahead in your Carb Cycling journey. Cheers to embracing a healthier lifestyle with carb cycling!

I sincerely hope that this book, which I worked so hard on, spoke to you. If you've enjoyed the journey, please consider leaving a review on Amazon. Your feedback not only helps me, but it also helps others discover this work.

Scan here to leave a review.

Index

Keto Cheesecake Bites; 56

Keto Chia Seed Pudding; 25

Keto Chocolate Avocado Mousse; 53

Keto Crab Cakes; 38

Keto Deviled Eggs; 60

Keto Egg Salad Lettuce Wraps; 27

Keto Portobello Mushroom Pizzas; 48

Lemon Blueberry Muffins; 92

Lemon Butter Asparagus Risotto; 82

Lemon Dill Baked Cod with Couscous; 77

Lemon Garlic Butter Baked Salmon; 34

Lemon Garlic Butter Shrimp with Linguine; 73

Lemon Herb Chicken with Roasted Potatoes; 72

Lemon Herb Grilled Steak; 31

Lentil and Vegetable Stew with Quinoa; 86

Lentil and Vegetable Stir-Fry with Brown Rice; 88

Low-Carb Chicken and Vegetable Stir-Fry; 45

Mediterranean Couscous Salad; 90

Mediterranean Tuna Salad with Orzo; 80

Mediterranean Zucchini Boats; 52

Mexican Cauliflower Rice; 42

Mixed Berry Crisp with Oat Topping; 91

Orange Glazed Chicken with Sweet Potatoes; 68

Orange Glazed Pound Cake; 94

Parmesan Crisps; 58

Peanut Butter and Banana Sandwich; 97

Peanut Butter Banana Breakfast Wrap; 67

Pork and Pineapple Skewers with Coconut Rice; 71

Pork Tenderloin with Dijon Mustard Glaze; 30

Pumpkin and Sage Pasta with Parmesan; 91

Pumpkin Pie with Whipped Cream; 94

Quinoa and Black Bean Salad; 89

Raspberry Coconut Chia Seed Pudding; 58

Raspberry Lemonade with Fresh Mint; 98

Roasted Chickpeas with Paprika; 96

Roasted Vegetable and Hummus Wrap; 90

Rosemary Roasted Pork Loin; 32

Seafood Paella with Saffron Rice; 77

Shirataki Noodles with Alfredo Sauce; 41

Shrimp and Avocado Salad; 35

Shrimp and Broccoli Stir-Fry with Quinoa; 76

Shrimp and Vegetable Skewers with Wild Rice; 79

Smoked Salmon and Cream Cheese Roll-Ups; 26

Smoked Salmon Cucumber Bites; 39

Spaghetti Squash Primavera; 49

Spaghetti Squash with Meat Sauce; 44

Spanish Chickpea and Rice Stew; 85

Spicy Cilantro Lime Tilapia; 37

Spicy Ground Turkey Lettuce Wraps; 33

Spicy Roasted Chickpeas; 59

Spicy Sausage and Orzo Soup; 84

Spinach and Feta Omelet; 24

Spinach and Ricotta Stuffed Shells; 89

Spinach and Sausage Soup; 42

Stuffed Bell Peppers with Cauliflower Rice; 46

Sweet and Sour Meatballs with Quinoa; 70

Sweet Potato and Black Bean Burritos; 87

Sweet Potato Hash with Eggs; 64

Teriyaki Chicken Skewers with Jasmine Rice; 69

Teriyaki Glazed Salmon with Jasmine Rice; 78

Thai Coconut Curry Noodles with Shrimp; 83

Tomato Basil Risotto; 81

Trail Mix with Dried Fruits and Nuts; 95

Tropical Fruit Salad with Honey Drizzle; 66

Tuna and Brown Rice Casserole; 74

Tuna Salad Lettuce Wraps; 36

Turkey and Veggie Breakfast Skillet; 28

Vanilla Coconut Flour Mug Cake; 57

Vegetable Fried Rice with Tofu; 80

Whole Grain Pancakes with Maple Syrup; 63

Wild Rice and Chicken Casserole; 84

Zucchini and Cheese Muffins; 25

Zucchini and Tomato Bake; 47

Zucchini Noodles with Pesto and Shrimp; 38

20431760R00060